AF430907

PHYSICAL PHARMACY
PRACTICAL TEXT
Third Edition

PHYSICAL PHARMACY PRACTICAL TEXT

Third Edition

Guru Prasad Mohanta,
M. Pharm., Ph.D., FIC.
Professor
Department of Pharmacy
Annamalai University
Annamalai Nagar – 608 002
Tamil Nadu

Prabal Kumar Manna,
M. Pharm., Ph.D., FIC, FICS.
Professor and Head
Department of Pharmacy
Annamalai University
Annamalai Nagar – 608 002
Tamil Nadu

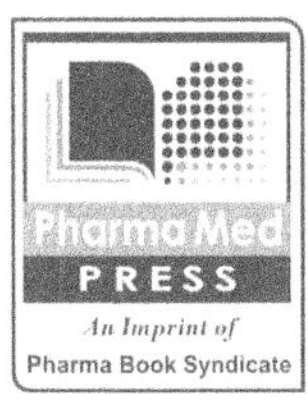

PharmaMed Press
An imprint of Pharma Book Syndicate
A unit of **BSP Books Pvt., Ltd.**
4-4-309/316, Giriraj Lane,
Sultan Bazar, Hyderabad - 500 095.

Physical Pharmacy Practical Text, Third Edition *by Guru Prasad Mohanta and Prabal Kumar Manna*

© 2017, 2012, 2006 *by Publisher*

Seventh Reprint 2019

Published by : **PharmaMed Press**

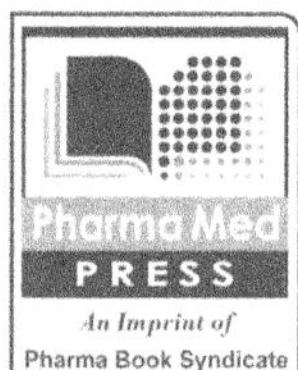

An imprint of Pharma Book Syndicate

A unit of BSP Books Pvt., Ltd.

4-4-309/316, Giriraj Lane, Sultan Bazar, Hyderabad - 500 095.
Phone: 040-23445688, 23445600; Fax: 91+40-23445611
E-mail: info@pharmamedpress.com
www.pharmamedpress.com/pharmamedpress.net

ISBN : 978-93-90211-00-5

PREFACE TO THIRD EDITION

"Perfection is not attainable, but if we chase perfection
we can catch excellence".

-Vince Lombardi

We have great pleasure in presenting the third edition of this practical text. We have been making attempt to make this text more acceptable to the students and the teachers. Perhaps we are successful to a reasonable extent making it flawless.

Like earlier editions, we strongly believe your feed-back for improving text would be our driving force. We look forward to your continuing patronage.

September 2016   **Guru Prasad Mohanta** [gpmohanta@hotmail.com]
                   Prabal Kumar Manna [pkmanna@rediffmail.com]

PREFACE TO FIRST EDITION

"The only person who has never made a mistake

the one who has never tried anything new in his lifetime"

-ALBERT EINSTEIN

The Physical Pharmacy subject and its principles provide a foundation to pharmacy students to understand the basis for development of new drugs, dosage forms and their improvement. Understanding the basic principles and developing skills and competency to perform physical pharmacy experiments is essential.

Looking at the need of pharmacy students, an attempt has been made to present the physical pharmacy experiments covering almost full requirements of various universities in a simple and understandable manner. Though it has been accepted to use only SI units in all scientific disciplines, pharmacy not being an exception, we are yet to completely transform to the new system of units. We have used the SI system of units in almost all experiments, but in some experiments conventional units are also mentioned for easy understanding the value.

Another important feature of this text is the "questions and answers portion" provided at the end of each experiment. This would help the students understanding the application of each experiment in pharmaceutical science and technology and prepare for the viva-voce, a component of practical examination.

The authors express their heartfelt thanks to Dr. R. Manavalan, Professor and Head, Department of Pharmacy of Annamalai University for his constant encouragement and help. They wish to acknowledge the support of their family members during preparing this manuscript. The permission to write this text from the authorities of Annamalai University is gratefully acknowledged. The authors express their sincere thanks to Mr. S. Selvamuthukumar, Lecturer in Pharmacy of Annamalai University, for drawing the illustrations for the book. The authors are thankful to M/S Pharma Book Syndicate, Hyderabad, for accepting to bring out the book in short notice.

The authors hope that the pharmacy students would find the text useful for performing Physical Pharmacy experiments and learning the concepts of physical pharmacy as they are applied to pharmaceutical sciences. The teachers too may find handy for training their students. Any suggestions and criticisms for improving the text would be gratefully accepted.

August 2006   *- Author*

CONTENTS

Chapter 10

Buffer 42

Chapter 11

Micromeritics 49

Chapter 12

Viscosity 63

Chapter 13

Adsorption Isotherm 67

Chapter 14

Physical Stability of Suspension 72

Chapter 15

Physical Stability of Emulsion 76

Chapter 16

Complexation 80

1

SI Systems of Units

The International System of Units (Systeme Internationale d' Units, SI) is the accepted system of measurement in all scientific fields including pharmacy. It is the developed version of metric system. However, still we find the use of many common units in the measurement. For the benefit of readers/students in the following table a conversion factor is given for converting the commonly used units in physical pharmacy experiments into SI units.

Physical Quantity	Commonly Used Unit	SI Unit	Conversion Factor (to be multiplied with)
Mass	g (gram)	kg (kilogram)	10^{-3}
Length	m (meter)	m (meter)	----------
Time	Minute	s (second)	60
Amount of substance	----------	mol (mole)	----------
Area	cm^2 (square centimeter)	m^2 (square meter)	10^{-4}
Volume	cc (cubic centimeter)	m^3 (cubic meter)	10^{-6}
Density	g/cc	kg / m^3 (kilogram per cubic meter)	10^3
Concentration	----------	mol/ m^3	----------
Force	dyn (dyne) = g cm/s^2	N (newton) = kg.m/s^2	10^{-5}
Pressure	dyn/ cm^2	Pa (pascal) = N/ m^2	10^{-1}
Dynamic viscosity	poise (dyn. cm^{-2}. second)	Pa.s (pascal.second)	10^{-1}
Kinematic viscosity	----------	m^2/s (square meter per second)	----------
Surface tension	dyn/cm	N/m (newton per meter)	10^{-3}
Temperature	°C	kelvin	+ 273.16 (here, it is to be added)

2

Solubility

Solubility is the measure of ability of a solute to get dissolved in a solvent. In other words, it is the measure of capacity of a solvent to dissolve a solute.

Mathematically it is expressed as the concentration of solute in a solution, which is in equilibrium with the solute (solid). That means the concentration of solute in a saturated solution is its solubility.

Though concentration can be expressed in many units, the solubility of solids in solvents is usually expressed in relation to solute and solvent that make a saturated solution. The pharmacopoeial expression of solubility is the number of milliliter of solvent in which 1 gram of solute will dissolve to make a saturated solution. When the exact solubility has not been determined, the solubility may be expressed in descriptive terms :

Descriptive terms	Parts of solvent required for 1 part of solute
Very soluble	Less than 1 part
Freely soluble	From 1 to 10 parts
Soluble	From 10 to 30 parts
Sparingly soluble	From 30 to 100 parts
Slightly soluble	From 100 to 1000 parts
Very slightly soluble	From 1000 to 10,000 parts
Insoluble/practically insoluble	More than 10,000 parts

The simplest way of solubility determination is to determine the concentration of solute in a saturated solution and work out the quantity of solvent in volume and quantity of solute in weight to express solubility.

The concentration can be determined by gravimetric, titrimetric or by any instrumental method of analysis.

2.1   Determination of Solubility by Gravimetric Method

Aim : To determine the solubility of Sodium Chloride in water (gravimetric method of estimation).

Principle : Mathematically solubility is expressed as the concentration of solute in a solution, which is in equilibrium with the solute (solid). That means the concentration of solute in a saturated solution is its solubility.

Though concentration can be expressed in many units, the solubility of solids in solvents is usually expressed in relation to solute and solvent that make a saturated solution. The pharmacopoeial expression of solubility is the number of milliliter of solvent in which 1 gram of solute will dissolve to make a saturated solution.

The simplest way of solubility determination is to determine the concentration of solute in a saturated solution and work out the quantity of solvent in volume and quantity of solute in weight to express solubility.

The concentration can be determined by gravimetric, titrimetric or by any instrumental method of analysis.

Sodium chloride can be estimated by simple gravimetric method.

Apparatus and Materials Required : Conical flask, weighing balance, evaporating dish, pipette, sodium chloride and water.

Process :

(i)   An increasing amount of sodium chloride is added to about 50 ml water in a conical flask with shaking until the solution is saturated and a part of solid is left undissolved (around 20 gram sodium chloride is required).

(ii)   The solution is filtered and 10 ml of the filtrate is pipetted out into a tared (preweighed) evaporating dish.

(iii) The dish containing 10 ml filtrate is weighed.

(iv)   The filtrate is evaporated to dryness and further dried at about 100 °C in an oven. Then it is cooled and weighed. Drying is continued till a constant weight is obtained.

Observation :   Room Temperature : _________°C

(i)   Weight of empty dish in g : w_1

(ii)   Weight of dish + 10 ml solution in g : w_2

(iii) Weight of dish + dry solution in g : w_3

Calculation :

Weight of solute in 10 ml solution in g $= w_3 - w_1$

Weight of solvent in 10 ml solution in g $= w_2 - w_3$

$$\text{Volume of solvent in ml} = \frac{\text{Weight of solvent}}{\text{Density of solvent (water)}} = \frac{w_2 - w_3}{\text{Density of water}}$$

Density of water at room temperature can be referred from the appendix (for rough calculation density of water may be considered as 1 g/ml).

Solubility is the parts of solvent required for 1 part of solute.

$(w_3 - w_1)$ g of solute requires $\dfrac{\left(w_2 - w_3\right)}{\text{Density of water}}$ ml of water.

1 g of solute will require $\dfrac{\left(w_2 - w_3\right)}{\left(w_3 - w_1\right)\text{Density of water}}$ ml of water.

Report : The solubility of Sodium Chloride in water at room temperature (specify) is 1 in ________ml. (the solubility of sodium chloride is 1 in 2.8 ml water at 25 °C)

Questions and Answers

1. How do you know that a saturated solution is prepared?

   Ans : While shaking excess solute in solvent, concentration is measured at frequent intervals. If two consecutive observations show the same concentration, it may be concluded that a saturated solution is prepared.

2. What is the need of mentioning temperature in expressing solubility?

   Ans : Solubility depends on temperature and pressure; and the solubility differs at different temperatures. It may either increase or decrease with rise of temperature depending on endothermic or exothermic dissolution.

3. How can solubility at higher or lower temperature be determined?

   Ans : For determination of solubility at higher temperature, the solvent is maintained at that temperature by keeping the container of solvent in a thermostatic water (or a suitable liquid) bath.

   For lower temperature, the conical flask containing saturated solution, prepared at room temperature, may be kept surrounded by ice-cold water to bring down the temperature to a desired level below that of environment. The temperature may be lowered continuously by adding small but increasing quantity of ice to the cooling bath.

Then solubility at that particular temperature can be determined in the usual way.

4. What is the importance of solubility in Pharmacy?

Ans : Solubility data help in the selection of solvent system for making liquid medicines. In case of insolubility or low solubility, the solubilization techniques are used to dissolve solid in water, or it may be made into a suspension.

Solubility less than 1 g/ml indicates the need of a salt form of the compound, if formulated as tablets or capsules in order to improve absorption.

Aqueous solubility less than 1% indicates the problem in absorption from oral administration.

2.2   Determination of Solubility by Titrimetry

Aim : To determine the solubility of Oxalic Acid in water (titrimetric method of estimation).

Principle : Same as described in the previous experiment.

In this case, the concentration of oxalic acid in the saturated solution is estimated by titrimetric method using standard sodium hydroxide solution.

Apparatus and Materials required : Conical flask, pipettes, burette, std. sodium hydroxide solution, oxalic acid, phenolphthalein and water.

Process :

(i)   An increasing amount of oxalic acid is added to about 50 ml water in a conical flask with shaking until the solution is saturated and a part of solid is left undissolved (around 08 gram oxalic acid is required).

(ii)   The solution is filtered and 10 ml of the filtrate is pipetted out into a conical flask and titrated against standard N/10 sodium hydroxide solution. Three observations are taken.

(iii)   The concentration of oxalic acid is determined from the titre value.

(iv)   The density of the filtrate is determined using a pycnometer.

Observation :   Room Temperature : _________ °C

Titration of oxalic acid solution with std. sodium hydroxide

No. of Observation	Volume of saturated solution of oxalic acid in ml	Burette Reading of Sodium hydroxide Solution in ml (Titre value)			Average volume of sodium hydroxide in ml
		Initial	Final	Difference	
1.					
2.					
3.					

Calculation :

Amount of oxalic acid present in 10 ml of saturated solution

$$= \frac{\text{Titre value} \times \text{Strength of sodium hydroxide solution in normality} \times \text{Equivalent factor}}{0.1} = w \text{ g}$$

The equivalent factor is 0.0063 (1 ml of N/10 sodium hydroxide solution is equivalent to 0.0063 g of oxalic acid)

Density of saturated solution $= x$ g/ml.

Density of water at room temperature can be referred from the appendix (for rough calculation density of water may be considered as 1 g/ml).

Volume of solvent (water) present in 10 ml saturated solution

$$= \frac{\text{Weight of solvent (water)}}{\text{Density of water}} = \frac{10\,x - w}{\text{Density of water}} \text{ ml.}$$

Therefore, Solubility in terms of number of ml of solvent required for 1 part of solute:

$$w \text{ g of solute requires } \frac{10\,x - w}{\text{Density of water}} \text{ ml of water.}$$

$$1 \text{ g of solute will require } \frac{10\,x - w}{\text{Density of water} \times w} \text{ ml of water.}$$

Report : The solubility of oxalic acid in water at room temperature (specify) is 1 in _______ ml.

(*Note :* the solubility of oxalic acid is 1 g in 7 ml water)

3

Distribution Coefficient

3.1 Determination of Distribution Coefficient without Association/Dissociation

Aim : To determine the distribution coefficient of iodine between carbon tetrachloride and water.

Principle : When a dissolved solid is distributed between two immiscible liquids/solvents, the ratio in which it distributes is called distribution coefficient or partition coefficient. If the solute is in same molecular condition in both the solvents, the distribution coefficient is constant and is dependent on temperature. This is also known as partition coefficient.

When a substance is distributed between two immiscible solvents: A and B,

$$\text{the distribution coefficient} = \frac{\text{Concentration of substance in A}}{\text{Concentration of substance in B}}$$

In pharmaceutical sciences, the organic solvent and water system is important.

The distribution or partition coefficient can be expressed as between organic phase and water, or between water and organic phase.

Though concentration of substance in organic and water phase needs to be mentioned in molar concentration; as distribution coefficient is a ratio term, the units get nullified. The concentration can thus be expressed in any unit, if the solute is in the same molecular state in both the phases.

The molecular state of iodine in both the solvents: carbon tetrachloride and water is same.

Apparatus and Materials required : Stoppered bottles, carbon tetrachloride, water, iodine, std. N/10 sodium thiosulphate, std. N/100 Sodium thiosulphate solution, potassium iodide, starch, pipettes and burettes.

Process :

I.   Distribution of Iodine in two phases :

1. A nearly saturated solution of iodine in 150 ml carbon tetrachloride is prepared in a beaker by adding few crystals of iodine to carbon tetrachloride and stirring with a glass rod.

2. The following mixtures of iodine solution in carbon tetrachloride and water are prepared in three glass-stoppered bottles :

Bottle number	Volume of pure carbon tetrachloride, ml	Volume of iodine solution in carbon tetrachloride, ml	Volume of water, ml
1.	20	0	200
2.	15	05	200
3.	10	10	200

3. After tightening the stopper, the bottles are shaken vigorously for few hours. At frequent intervals of 1 to 2 minutes the stoppers are removed to release pressure.

4. The bottles are then kept undisturbed allowing the liquids to separate into two layers. The lower layer is carbon tetrachloride and the upper one is that of water.

   (*Note :* The separating funnels can also be used in place of glass stoppered bottles.)

II.   The determination of concentration of Iodine in two phases :

1. 50 ml of aqueous layer is pipetted out from first bottle into a conical flask containing about 5 ml 10% potassium iodide solution and 1 ml starch solution (taking care that the tip of the pipette is above the interface in order to prevent any carbon tetrachloride getting into the pipette). It is then titrated against N/100 sodium thiosulphate solution. The end point of titration: disapperance of blue colour of starch – iodine complex.

   Similarly 50 ml quantities of aqueous layer are withdrawn from other bottles and titrated.

2. 5 ml of carbon tetrachloride layer is pipetted out into a conical flask containing 20 ml of 10% potassium iodide solution and 1 ml starch solution as indicator. It is then titrated against std. N/10 sodium thiosulphate. The end point of titration: disapperance of blue colour of starch – iodine complex.

   (While titrating the organic layer (carbon tetrachloride), the titration flask must be shaken continuously to allow intimate mixing for quick reaction between iodine and thiosulphate.)

   Similarly 5 ml of carbon tetrachloride layer is withdrawn from other bottles and titrated.

Bottle number	Volume of N/100 sodium thiosulaphate for 50 ml aqueous layer (ml)	Concentration of iodine in aqueous layer (molarity)	Volume of N/10 sodium thiosulaphate for 5 ml carbon tetrachloride layer (ml)	Concentration of iodine in carbon tetrachloride layer (molarity)	Distribution coefficient	Average value
1.						
2.						
3.						

Observation and Calculation :   Room temperature : _________ ºC.

(1ml of N/10 sodium thiosulphate is equivalent to 0.5×10^{-4} g mole Iodine.)

Report : The distribution coefficient of iodine between carbon tetrachloride and water is _________ at _______ ºC.

(The distribution coefficient of iodine between carbon tetrachloride and water at 25 ºC is 83.3 and the same between water and carbon tetrachloride 0.012.)

Questions and Answers

1. What is the relationship between solubility and distribution coefficient?

    Ans : In sparingly soluble substances and when the solute is in same molecular condition (no dissociation or association), then distribution coefficient is approximately equal to the ratio of solubility in the respective solvents.

2. What is the need of potassium iodide solution in the titration?

    Ans : The addition of aqueous potassium iodide solution facilitates extraction of iodine into the aqueous solution during titration due to the formation of unstable complex ion

    $$I_3^- \text{ as } K^+ + I^- + I_2 \Leftrightarrow K^+ + I_3^-$$

3. How can the distribution coefficient be determined when association or dissociation of solute takes place in either of solvent?

    Ans : Please refer the next experiment where determination of distribution coefficient of benzoic acid between benzene and water is discussed.

4. Does the distribution coefficient depend on the total amount solid dissolved?

    Ans : No. It is independent of amount of solid dissolved. This is evident from the experiment just performed where concentration of iodine is different in different bottles, but distribution coefficient remains same.

5. What are the importances of partition coefficient in pharmacy?

   Ans :

   (i)   The rate of release of medicaments from dosage forms like suppositories and ointments is dependent on the partition coefficient of drug between the base and body fluid. Quick release causes quick action. Slow release delays action but prolongs it.

   (ii) The absorption of drugs from gastro intestinal tract (GIT), distribution to various tissues depends on the partition coefficient of drug between lipoidal layer (cell membrane) and aqueous body fluids.

   (iii) Partition coefficient of preservatives between bacterial cells and the surrounding aqueous medium is determining factor for their effectiveness.

   (iv) In preserving the emulsion system, the distribution of preservatives preferentially to aqueous fluid is preferred as microbes normally grow only in aqueous phase.

   (v)   The principle of partition chromatography (a separation and analytical technique) is based on the difference in partition coefficient of components to be separated between two immiscible liquids or between a liquid and vapour phase.

   (vi) It also helps in calculating the volume of solvents required for extraction.

3.2   Determination of Distribution Coefficient Involving Association

Aim : To determine the distribution coefficient (partition coefficient) of benzoic acid between benzene and water.

Principle : If the solute exists in same molecular state in both solvents, the simple concentration ratio of the solute in solvents represents the constant, distribution coefficient.

However, if, in one solvent, the solute exists as normal molecular species while in other it is associated or dissociated, then the simple concentration ratio is no longer constant.

If association occurs in one phase and n molecules of the solute combine together to form a complex molecule; then the distribution coefficient calculation the nth root of concentration of associated form is used.

Benzoic acid exists in water as monomer and in benzene as dimer (association). The concentration ratio between water and benzene can be written as $\dfrac{\text{Concentration in water}}{\sqrt{\text{Concentration in benzene}}}$ and similarly the ratio between benzene and water would be $\dfrac{\sqrt{\text{Concentration in benzene}}}{\text{concentration in water}}$. This ratio is partition coefficient and constant.

Apparatus and Materials required : Stoppered glass bottles, benzoic acid, benzene, N/10 sodium hydroxide solution, phenolphthalein indicator, pipettes and burettes.

Process :

(i) About 1, 2 and 3 g quantities of benzoic acid are transferred into three labeled stoppered glass bottles.

(ii) Around 50 ml of benzene and around 50 ml of water are added to each bottle.

(iii) After tightly stopping the bottles, they are vigorously shaken every 3 to 5 minutes for about one hour. The stoppers are removed to release the pressure.

(iv) The bottles are then kept undisturbed to get the layers separated. The lower layer is aqueous and upper layer is organic (benzene).

(The separating funnels may be used instead of stoppered glass bottles).

(v) 10 ml of the benzene layer is pipetted out into a conical flask containing around 30 ml water. The solution is then titrated against N/10 sodium hydroxide using phenolphthalein as indicator. (During titration the contents should be shaken vigorously to ensure rapid and complete extraction of benzoic acid from benzene).

Similarly 10 ml benzene layer of other bottles are also titrated.

(vi) 10 ml of aqueous layer is pipetted out into a conical flask and titrated against N/50 sodium hydroxide using phenolphthalein as indicator.

Similarly 10 ml of aqueous layer of other bottles are also titrated.

Observation and Calculation :

Room temperature : ________ °C.

Bottle no.	Volume of N/50 sodium hydroxide for 10 ml aqueous layer (ml)	Concentration of benzoic acid in aqueous layer (Molarity)	Volume of N/10 sodium hydroxide for 10 ml benzene layer (ml)	Conc. of benzoic acid in benzene layer (Molarity)	$\dfrac{\text{Concentration in organic phase}}{\text{Concentration in aqueous phase}}$	$\sqrt{\dfrac{\text{concentration in benzene}}{\text{concentration in water}}}$
1.						
2.						
3.						

Normality and Molarity of benzoic acid is same.

The concentration in Normality can be obtained from the relationship:

$$S_1 \times V_1 = S_2 \times V_2$$

where S_1 and V_1 are strength in Normality and volume in ml of sodium hydroxide; and S_2 and V_2 are strength in Normality and volume in ml of benzoic acid.

(1 Normal sodium hydroxide $\equiv$ 1 Normal benzoic acid)

Report : The distribution coefficient of benzoic acid between benzene and water is _______ at _______ °C.

(The distribution coefficient of benzoic acid between benzene and water at 25°C is around 38.)

Questions and Answers

1. What do you know that the solute is in same molecular concentration or associated or dissociated?

   Ans : If the concentration ratio does not vary with change in concentration of solute and remains constant, then it is understandable that the solute exists in same molecular species. On the other hand, variation in concentration ratio with change in concentration of solute indicates either association or dissociation.

   In the present exercise, it is noticed that ratio of concentration of benzoic acid in benzene and water varies in different bottles (having different benzoic acid concentration).

2. How can one know that the benzoic acid is associated and exists as dimmer in benzene?

   Ans : The logarithmic plot: Log concentration (organic phase) in X-axis and Log concentration (aqueous phase) in Y-axis produces a straight line. The value of n (number of molecules associated) and distribution coefficient can be determined from this curve where 1/n is the slope and –log (distribution coefficient) is the intercept in Y-axis.

4

Density

4.1 Determination of Density

Aim : To determine the density of zinc oxide by liquid displacement method.

Principle : The density is weight per unit volume. For solids, it is determined pycnometrically from the liquid displaced by the submerged solid. When a solid mass is immersed in a liquid in which it is insoluble, it will displace equal volume of liquid. That is,

$$\text{volume of solid mass} = \text{volume of displaced liquid.}$$

Apparatus and Materials required : Pycnometer (specific gravity bottle), zinc oxide, water

Process :

    (i) About 1 g of material (zinc oxide) is filled into a dried and tared (pre weighed) specific gravity bottle and weighed.

    (ii) The specific gravity bottle containing zinc oxide is filled with water and weighed.

    (iii) After cleaning, the same specific gravity bottle is filled with water and weighed.

Observation :

Room Temperature : ______ °C

Weight of empty dry specific gravity bottle = a g

Weight bottle containing around 1 g of zinc oxide = c g

Weight of bottle containing zinc oxide and filled with water = d g

Weight of bottle filled with water = b g

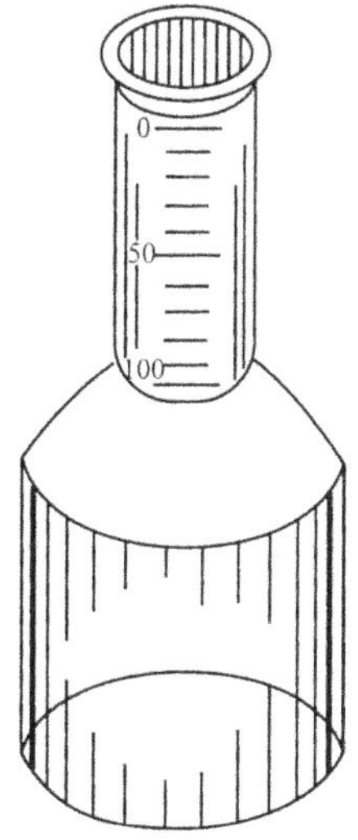

Calculation : $\text{Density} = \dfrac{\text{Mass of solid}}{\text{Mass of displaced liquid} \div \text{Density of liquid}}$

Mass of solid = (c - a) g

Mass of displaced liquid = mass of total liquid – mass of volume of liquid present with the solid = (b - a) – (d - c)

$\therefore \text{ Density} = \dfrac{c - a}{(b - a) - (d - c)} \times \text{density of water} = \underline{\qquad} \text{ g/ml.}$

Density of water at room temperature can be referred from the table in the appendix.

Multiply the density value in g/ml with 10^3 to get the density in SI unit: kg/m^3

Report : The density of zinc oxide is _______ kg/m^3 at temperature ___ ^{o}C.

(Density of few solids in g/ml :   Calcium oxide : 3.3

Zinc oxide : 5.6

Sodium chloride : 2.16

Kaolin : 2.2 to 2.5)

Questions and Answers

1. What criteria should be used in the selection of liquid for density measurement of solids?

    Ans : Solids should be insoluble in the liquid and heavier than it.

2. What are the importances of solid density?

    Ans :

    (i)   It is the characteristic of the compound.

    (ii) Density is an important criterion in packing. Denser particles get closer packing with reduced porosity.

    (iii) Density of solids in suspension is a rate-controlling factor in settling.

    Stoke's law :

$\text{Rate of settling} = \dfrac{\text{diameter}^2 \times \text{Density differnce between solid and liquid} \times g}{18 \times \text{Viscosity of liquid}}$

The rate of settling can be minimized by reducing the density difference between solid and liquid phase.

(iv) Density is an important consideration in the formulation of powder insufflations, where the patient has to inhale a fine powder directly into lungs.

(v) Knowledge of powder properties including that of density is essential for designing and satisfactory operation of pneumatic conveyer system.

3. What are the other methods of determination of density?

   Ans : If the material is porous, a helium densitometer is used. This is a better method as it gives more accurate results because helium can penetrate into smallest pores than water.

4. How can you determine the density of liquids?

   Ans : As specific gravity bottle has fixed volume, it can be filled with the liquid and the weight of filled liquid can be determined from the difference in weight of empty and filled bottle. Then this figure is divided by the volume of the liquid (capacity of specific gravity bottle).

5

Bulk Density

5.1   Determination of Bulk Density

Aim : To determine the bulk density of magnesium carbonate.

Principle : Bulk density is the mass of a powder divided by the bulk volume.

$$\text{Bulk density} = \frac{\text{Mass of powder}}{\text{Bulk volume}}$$

Apparatus and materials : Measuring cylinder, magnesium carbonate and weighing balance.

Process :

    (i)   The powder whose bulk density is to be determined is passed through sieve no. 20.

    (ii) About 20 g is weighed accurately and carefully introduced into a 100 ml graduated measuring cylinder.

    (iii) The cylinder is dropped at 2-seconds interval onto a hard surface three times from a height of 1 inch.

    (iv) The volume of powder is noted.

Observation and Calculation : Weight of powder = W_1 g

Volume of powder = V cc

$$\text{The bulk density} = \frac{\text{Mass of Powder}}{\text{Bulk Volume of powder}} = \frac{W_1}{V}\ g/cc$$

(convert the value to SI units by multiplying by a factor 10^3)

Report : The bulk density of magnesium carbonate is _______ kg/m^3.

Questions and Answers

1. Which value is higher – true density or bulk density, for a substance?

   Ans : True density is higher as the true volume is lower than bulk volume.

2. What is the difference between light and heavy magnesium carbonate?

   Ans : The light means low bulk density or larger bulk volume and similarly the heavy means high bulk density or smaller bulk volume. These terms have no relation to true densities.

3. What are the applications of bulk density?

   Ans :

   (i)   It offers valuable information on tablet porosity and its relation to tablet hardness and disintegration.

   (ii) As a characteristic, it is used as indicator for uniformity checking of bulk chemicals. Bulk density and tapped density are mandatory specification [US FDA].

   (iii) It is an important consideration in packing of powders. The bulk density of calcium carbonate may vary from 0.1 to 1.3. This indicates that depending on variety, light variety would require a container of size that is 13 times larger than required for heavy one.

6

Specific Gravity

6.1 Determination of Specific Gravity

Aim : To determine the specific gravity of glycerin.

Principle : Specific gravity is the ratio of the density of a substance to the density of water. The density of both the substances should be recorded at the same temperature unless specified. It is also called relative density. It is often defined as the ratio of mass of a substance to the mass of an equal volume of water at 4 °C or at some specified temperature.

$$\frac{\text{Density of subsatnce}}{\text{Density of water}} = \frac{\text{mass of subsatnce/volume}}{\text{mass of water/volume}}$$

When volume is equal, specific gravity is the ratio of weight of liquid to the weight of equal volume of water.

Apparatus and materials required : Pycnometer (specific gravity bottle), glycerin, water and weighing balance.

Process :

(i) The clean and dry empty specific bottle is weighed.

(ii) Then the bottle is completely filled with distilled water and weighed.

(iii) After cleaning and drying, the bottle is filled completely with the liquid whose specific gravity is to be determined (glycerin) and weighed.

Observation :   Room Temperature : _______ °C

Weight of empty dry specific gravity bottle = w_1 g

Weight of specific gravity bottle filled with water = w_2 g

Weight of specific gravity bottle filled with glycerin = w_3 g

Calculation :

Mass of water $= (w_2 - w_1)$ g

Mass of liquid $= (w_3 - w_1)$ g

$$\text{Specific gravity} = \frac{\text{mass of liquid}}{\text{mass of equal volume of water}} = \frac{w_3 - w_1}{w_2 - w_1}$$

Report : The specific gravity of glycerin is ___________ at ___________ °C.

(The specific gravity of glycerin is 1.16)

Specific gravity of few liquids (Values Are Approximate).

Ethy alcohol	0.79
Acetic acid	1.05
Chloroform	1.49
Ethyl acetate	0.90
Castor oil	0.97
Olive oil	0.92

Questions and Answers

1. What is the unit of specific gravity?

   Ans : Specific gravity is a ratio term between two densities and thus this is a dimensionless number. It has no unit.

2. What are the other methods of determination of specific gravity?

   Ans : This can be determined by use of Mohr-Westphal balance or hydrometer.

3. How can the density be determined from the specific gravity?

   Ans : Multiplication of specific gravity by the density of water at that temperature yields the density of the liquid.

4. What is the application of specific gravity in pharmacy?

   Ans : Liquids are easier to measure than weighing. The specific gravity figure can be utilized to calculate the density (or weight per ml) of liquid substance. The weight can be converted to volume and volume equivalent to weight can be easily measured.

7

Flow Properties

7.1 Determination of Flow Properties of Powders by Angle of Repose

Aim : To study the flow properties of powders/granules (potassium dichromate/ some granules) by determination of angle of repose.

Principle : When a powder material passes through an orifice, they are called free flowing; while those do not pass even though the particles are very much smaller than orifice, are called cohesive. Angle of repose is one of the simplest techniques used to determine the flowability of powder materials.

The angle of repose is defined as the angle of elevation to the horizontal at which the powder commences to slide upon itself. When an open-ended cylinder containing powder with the bottom resting on the horizontal surface, is lifted vertically, the powder will form a heap. The angle of conical heap can be 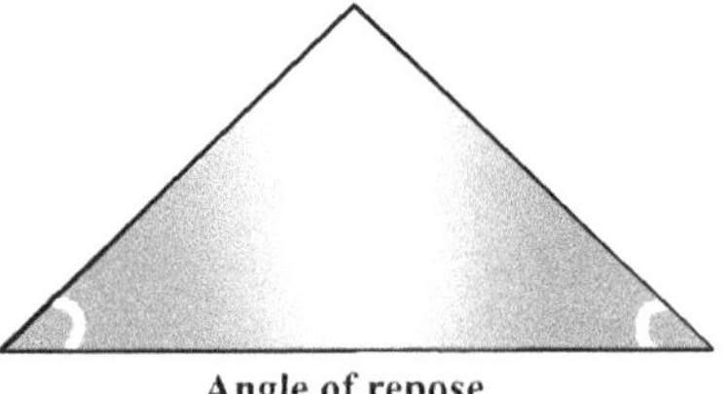

Angle of repose

determined from the diameter or radius of the base and height of the cone. $\tan \theta = \text{height/radius}$; thus $\theta = \tan^{-1} (\text{height/radius})$.

The high value of θ is the indication of cohesive nature of powder and low value for free flowing. When the angle is at minimum i.e., $25°$, the powders will flow easily.

Apparatus and materials required : open ended cylinder, scale, graph paper and powder sample (s) (potassium dichromate/some granules)

Process :

(i)   The powder is filled into an open-ended cylinder with the bottom resting on a horizontal surface.

(ii) The cylinder is then lifted vertically allowing the powder to form a heap on the horizontal.

(iii) The diameter of the base of the cone is determined by measuring the same in more than one direction. The radius is calculated from the diameter.

(iv) The height of the heap is also measured.

The experiment is repeated at least three times for each sample.

Observation and calculation :

Sample :

Number of observation	Height of heap in cm	Average height in cm.	Radius of the base of the cone in cm.	Average radius of the base of the cone in cm.	tan θ	θ
1.						
2.						
3.						

Report : The powder is free flowing/not free flowing as the angle of repose is close to 25°/more than 30°. (The report can also be written as excellent/good/passable/very poor flow based an angle of repose).

Questions and Answers

1. What are the other methods of determining angle of repose?

    Ans : The angle of repose can be determined from the heap formed by allowing the material to flow through a funnel, secured firmly in a stand, onto a horizontal surface beneath. But it has some limitations (suitable for free flowing powders only and does not produce reproducible results.)

2. How can you predict the flowability from the angle of repose?

    Ans :

Angle of repose in ^{0}	Type of flow
< 25	Excellent
25 – 30	Good
30 – 40	Passable
> 40	Very poor

3. What are the factors that influence the flowability of powders?

    Ans :

    (i) ***Shape of particles :*** Spherical particles flow easily and uniformly compared to irregular and other shaped particles. Granules flow better than powders.

    (ii) ***Size of the particles :*** Very small particles (less than 10mm) will have poor flow. Increase in particle size improves flowabilty and after maximum flow rate, further increase in size decreases the flow rate as size of the particles approach that of orifice.

    Removal of the fines from the powders increases flowability.

    (iii) ***Moisture content :*** Moisture makes the powder mass damp and (decreases) flowability. The drying of powders improves flowability by removing moisture.

4. What are significances of flow property of powders in Pharmacy?

    Ans : The tablets or capsules manufactured in one batch (also in batch to batch) should contain uniform quantity of medicament (s) that in turn determine their weight. The fill weight depends on the flow of powders (formulation mixture)/ granules. The poor flow is likely to result with less fill weight (in turn less quantity of medicament). The tablets/capsules will fail to comply with uniformity of weight requirements.

7A

Carr's Index

7A.1 Determination of Flow Properties of Powders by Carr's Index

Aim : To determine the flow properties of powders/granules (by determining the carr's index/bulk density).

Principle : The flowability is related to carr's index. The carr's index is described as

$$\% = \frac{\text{Tapped density-Poured density}}{\text{Tapped density}} \times 100$$

The lower the carr's index, better the flow.

Apparatus and materials required : Same as that described under bulk density experiment.

Process : Determination of tapped density and poured density:

(i) A fixed quantity of powder is poured into a measuring cylinder and the volume is noted. This figure is used for calculating poured density.

(ii) The tapped density is then determined as described under bulk density determination experiment (tapped density and bulk density are same).

Observation and Calculation :

Poured density determination : Weight of powder = W_1 g

Volume of powder = V_1 cc

Bulk density determination : Weight of powder $= W_2$ g

$$\text{Volume of powder} = V_2 \text{ cc}$$

$$\text{The bulk density} = \frac{\text{Mass of powder}}{\text{Bulk Volume of powder}} = \frac{W_2}{V_2} \text{ g/cc}$$

$$\text{Carr's index (\%)} \ \frac{\text{Tapped density-poured density}}{\text{Tapped density}} \times 100$$

The carr's index of _______ is _______ .

Report : The flow property of powder is excellent/good/fair/poor.

Questions and Answers

1. How is carr's index related to flow property?

   Ans :

Carr's index	Type of flow
5 – 15	Excellent
13 – 16	Good
18 – 21	Fair to Passable*
23 – 35	Poor*
33 – 38	Very Poor
>40	Extremely poor

* The flow property can be improved by adding flow improving agent (glidant).

2. How is compressibility index related to flow property?

   Ans: The percentage compressibility can be calculated as:

$$\% \text{Compressibility} = \frac{\text{Tapped density} - \text{Poured density}}{\text{Tapped density}} \times 100$$

The term compressibility is a misnomer as there is no compression involved. However, there is a close relationship between percent compressibility and flowability. 5-15% compressibility indicates excellent flow and % compressibility above 40 indicates extremely poor flow.

3. Is there any other index that gives idea on flow propety of powders?

   Ans: Yes, this is called Hausner Ratio.

$$\text{Hausner ratio} = \frac{\text{Tapped density}}{\text{Poured density}} \quad \text{Hausner ratio of less 1.25}$$

indicates good flow, while greater than 1.5 indicates poor flow.

8

Dissociation Constant (pK$_a$)

8.1   Determination of Dissociation Constant

Aim : To determine the dissociation constant (pK$_a$) of a weak acid (salicylic acid).

Principle : Weak acids and weak bases do not ionise completely in aqueous solutions like strong acids and bases. The degree of ionisation is expressed in terms of ionisation and dissociation constant, which is expressed conveniently in terms of pK$_a$ for both acids and bases. pK$_a$ is the negative logarithm of acid dissociation constant K$_a$ in the same way as pH is used to represent negative logarithm of hydronium ion concentration.

The dissociation constant value (pK$_a$) for weak acids or bases can be determined using Henderson - Hasselbalch equation:

$$pH = pK_a + \log \frac{[\text{ionized acid}]}{[\text{unionized acid}]} = pK_a + \log \frac{[\text{salt}]}{[\text{acid}]}$$

$$\text{or} \qquad pK_a = pH - \log \frac{[\text{ionized acid}]}{[\text{unionized acid}]}$$

At 50% neutralization point, that is when [ionised acid] = [unionized acid], the value of pK$_a$ = pH

The value of pK$_a$ can be directly measured by recording the pH at 50% neutralization point.

Materials and apparatus required : Salicylic acid, standard sodium hydroxide solution, pH meter, conical flask, burette, pipettes and indicator.

Procedure :

(i)   10 ml of 0.5%w/v solution of salicylic acid in methanol is pipetted out to a conical flask. (Should not be sucked by mouth as methanol is toxic; a bulb pipette should be used).

(ii)   This is then titrated against 0.5 N sodium hydroxide solution using methyl red as indicator to complete neutralization. The burette reading (consumption of sodium hydroxide) is noted.

(iii)   Similarly 10 ml of 0.5%w/v salicylic acid solution is taken into a flask and titrated against standard 0.5N sodium hydroxide solution to 50% neutralization point (that is, half of the sodium hydroxide consumed in previous titration is added).

(iv)   The pH of this half neutralized solution is recoded using a pH meter.

Observation and Calculation :   Room Temperature: __________ $^\circ$C.

Let, the volume of 0.5 N sodium hydroxide consumed in titration with 10 ml 0.5% salicylic acid solution (complete neutralization) = Lets say x ml.

Volume of 0.5 N sodium hydroxide solution required for half neutralization = x/2 ml.

The pH of half neutralization solution = __________ .

Report : The pK_a value of salicylic acid at __________ $^\circ$C is __________ .

   (the normal value is 2.97)

The pK_a value of some weak acids and bases :

Weak acids	Weak bases
Paracetamol : 9.92	Glycine : 2.35
Aspirin : 3.49	Atropine : 9.68
Benzoic acid : 4.2	Caffeine : 3.6 and 0.6
	Codeine : 0.82
	Urea : 0.18

Questions and Answers

1. What are the other methods of determination of dissociation constants?

   Ans : Conductometry and spectrophotometry. The spectrophotometric method too is based on Henderson-Hassselbalch equation. However, conductometric method requires knowledge of degree of ionisation.

2. What are the significances of pK$_a$ value?

   Ans : A low value of pK$_a$ (or, higher value of pK$_b$) is the characteristics of relatively strong acids or weak bases. Similarly high values of pK$_a$ (or, low values of pK$_b$) indicate relatively weak acids or strong bases.

   When the value of pK$_a$ is less than around 2, the acids are termed as strong acids. Similarly in case of base, when this value is around 12, the bases are termed as strong bases.

3. Does the dissociation constant get affected by temperature?

   Ans : Yes, it is dependent on temperature. Normally it increases with rise of temperature. The temperature needs to be recorded at the time of experiment.

4. What is the relation between pK$_a$ and pK$_b$?

   Ans : pK$_a$ + pK$_b$ = 14 at 25 °C.

   Once pK$_b$ for the base is determined, the pK$_a$ value can be calculated from the above equation. As pH is used to indicate the acidity and alkalinity, pK$_a$ can be used to express dissociation constant for both acids and bases.

5. What is the unit of dissociation constant?

   Ans : Dissociation constant, pK$_a$, has no unit.

6. What are the importances of pK$_a$ in pharmacy?

   Ans :

   (i) The degree of ionisation depends on the pH of environment. The degree of ionisation can be calculated from the equation:

   $$\text{Percentage of ionised molecule} = \frac{100}{1 + \dfrac{1}{\text{antilog}\,(pH - pK_a)}}$$

   Unionised portion is more lipid soluble and hence is better absorbed. Thus the portion of gastrointestinal tract (GIT), where drugs will predominantly be in unionised state, is a good site for absorption. Thus the acidic drugs are better absorbed from stomach than the intestine and the basic drugs are better absorbed from the intestine than stomach.

   (ii) Unionized molecules penetrate cell membranes (which are lipid in nature) more readily than ions. The increased antibacterial action of benzoic acid (preservative) is reflected in acidic solution.

9

Surface Tension

9.1 Determination of Hydrophilic-Lipophilic Balance (HLB) Number

Aim : To determine the HLB number of polyoxyethylene sorbitan monolaurate (Tween 20).

Principle : The hydrophilic-lipophilic balance (HLB) of a surfactant is a measure of its polarity. The HLB value of nonionic surfactant can be calculated using the formula :

$$HLB = 20 \left(1 - \frac{S}{A} \right)$$ where S is saponification number of ester and A is

acid number of fatty acid.

Apparatus and Materials required : Round bottom reflux, condenser, alcoholic potassium hydroxide, phenolphthalein, lauric acid, standard N/2 hydrochloric acid, and standard N/10 potassium hydroxide.

Process : It is restricted to the determination of saponification number and acid number.

A.   Determination of saponification number :

  (i) Around 1 gram of sample (Tween 20) is accurately weighed and transferred to round bottom flask. 30 ml alcoholic potassium hydroxide (2.82%) is added and refluxed on a boiling water bath for about 1 hour.

(ii)   A blank experiment is performed in the same way but without using the sample.

(iii)   The reaction mixtures are cooled down to room temperature and titrated against standard N/2 hydrochloric acid using phenolphthalein as indicator taking colour change from pink to colourless or slightly yellow as end point.

B.   Determination of acid number :

(i)   Around 500 mg of lauric acid is accurately weighed and mixed with 10 ml alcohol and 10 ml ether in a conical flask (slight warming may be necessary to dissolve lauric acid).

(ii)   The above mixture is titrated against standard N/10 potassium hydroxide using phenolphthalein as indicator.

Observation and Calculation :

Weight of sample taken for saponification number determination = ________ g.

Weight of sample taken for acid number determination = ________ g.

Determination of saponification number :

Let titre value of sample = V_1 ml.

Titre value of blank = V_2 ml.

$(V_2 - V_1)$ ml of N/2 hydrochloric acid equivalent potassium hydroxide is required to neutralize the taken sample.

$(V_2 - V_1)$ ml of N/2 hydrochloric acid $\equiv (V_2 - V_1)$ ml of N/2 Potassium hydroxide

1000 ml N Potassium hydroxide $\equiv$ 56000 mg of Potassium hydroxide

$$(V_2 - V_1) \text{ ml of N/2 Potassium hydroxide} \equiv 56000 \times \frac{N}{2} \times \frac{(V_2 - V_1)}{1000}$$

mg Potassium hydroxide

$$\text{Saponification number} = \left[56000 \times \frac{N}{2} \times \frac{(V_2 - V_1)}{1000} \right] \div \text{amount of sample in g}$$

Note : The **saponification number** is defined as number of mg of potassium hydroxide required to neutralize the acid present in one gram of substance.

Acid number is defined as the number of mg of potassium hydroxide required to neutralize the free acid present in one gram of substance.

This formula can be written in a simplified way :

$$\text{Saponification number (S)} = \frac{(V_2 - V_1) \times \text{Normality of hydrochloric acid} \times \text{Eq.Wt.of Potassium hydroxide}}{\text{Amount of sample in g}}$$

Determination of acid number :

Let the titre value of N/10 potassium hydroxide $= V_3$ ml.

V_3 ml of N/10 potassium hydroxide is required to neutralize the free acid in taken sample.

$$\text{Acid number (A)} = \frac{V_3 \times \text{Eq.Wt of Potassium hydroxide} \times \text{Normality of Potassium hydroxide}}{\text{weight of sample in g}}$$

$$HLB = 20(1-S/A)$$

Report : The HLB number of polyoxyethelene sorbitan monolaurate (tween 20) is __________. (the normal values: S = 45.5, A = 276 and HLB = 16.7)

Questions and Answers

1. What is the significance of HLB value?

   Ans : HLB value (scale), ranges from 1 to 40, is an indication of polarity. Higher the value, more polar is the surfactant (i.e. more hydrophilic). The spans are lipophilic (HLB values 1.8 to 8.6) and tweens are hydrophilic (HLB values more than 9.6).

   Surfactant functions on the basis of its HLB value :

Functions	HLB Value
Antifoaming	1 to 3
Emulsifying agent (w/o)	3 to 6
Wetting agents	7 to 9
Emulsifying agent (o/w)	8 to 18
Detergents	13 to 15
Solubilizing agents	15 to 20

2. What is the application of HLB value?

   Ans : In the HLB system, in addition to assigning values to emulsifying agents, values are also assigned to oils and oily substances. In the preparation of emulsion, emulsifying agent (s) having the same or nearly same HLB value as that of oily substance(s) of intended emulsion is selected. If necessary, a blend of emulsifying agents is used to get nearly desired HLB value.

3. What are the other methods of determination of HLB value?

   Ans : A method described by Davis assigns group numbers to the component groups of the surfactant molecule. By adding the group numbers of a surfactant, HLB value of that surfactant can be calculated from the equation :

   HLB = Σ(hydrophilic group number) - Σ(lipophilic group number) + 7

Example :	Hydrophilic group	Group number
	$-SO_3^-\ Na^+$	38.7
	Lipophilic group	Group number
	-CH-	0.475

9.2   Surface Tension

Molecules within the bulk of a liquid are subjected to attractive forces (*van der waals* force) equally in all directions, whereas those at the surface have very little attraction from the vapour and thus experience a net pull into the liquid. This net inward attraction causes the surface to be under tension called surface tension.

The surface tension (ST) is defined as the force acting within the surface in a direction normal (right angle) to a line of 1 m length. The unit is mNm^{-1} (milli Newton per meter).

In this chapter experiments involving determination of ST by drop weight method and drop count method using stalagmometer and determination of critical micelle concentration are discussed.

9.2.1 Determination of Surface Tension by Drop Weight Method

Aim : To determine the surface tension of a liquid (glycerin) using stalagmometer by drop weight method.

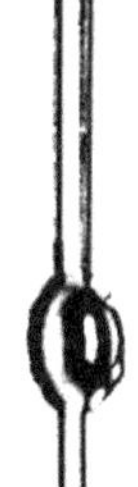

Principle :

The Surface tension (ST) measurement involves counting of number of drops formed when definite volume of liquid is allowed to flow slowly out of a capillary orifice (stalagmometer). The ratio of a weight (w_1) of a drop of the liquid to that of a reference substance (w_2) falling from the same capillary orifice is equal to the ratio of their surface tension.

The weight of the drop in mg of a test liquid, $w_1 = 2\pi r\gamma_1$.

Correction factor : The correction factor depends on the radius of tip, r and the cube root of volume of the drop.

The weight of drop of the reference liquid, $w_2 = 2\pi r\gamma_2$. correction factor (from the same capillary)

As the same apparatus is used for both the liquids, the correction factor is same assuming that the drop volumes are not different.

$$\frac{w_1}{w_2} = \frac{2\pi r\gamma_1.\text{correction factor}}{2\pi r\gamma_2.\text{correction factor}} = \frac{\gamma_1}{\gamma_2}$$

γ_1 and γ_2 are the surface tension of the test liquid and reference liquid respectively.

$$\gamma_1 = \frac{w_1}{w_2} \cdot \gamma_2$$

The value of ST of the liquid can be calculated by taking two observations: the weight of one drop of liquid and that of a reference liquid, if ST of the reference substance is known. Water is usually used as reference liquid.

Apparatus and materials required : Stalagmometer, glycerin, water, balance, weighing bottle.

Process :

    (i)   The cleaned stalagmometer is fixed with a clamp and filled with water by sucking.

    (ii)   Around 20-30 drops of water, falling from the stalagmometer is collected in a dry and tared (preweighed) weighing bottle, and weighed.

    (iii)   The stalagmometer is then dried and the experiment is repeated with the liquid whose ST is to be determined.

Care should be taken during experiment that the number of drops does not exceed 20 per minute.

Observation and Calculation :   Room temperature : _________ °C.

(i)   Weight of the clean and dry weighing bottle = x_1 g.

(ii)   Weight of the dry weighing bottle + 20 drops liquid = y_1 g.

(iii)   Weight of the clean and dry weighing bottle = x_1 g.

(iv)   Weight of the dry weighing bottle + 20 drops water = y_2 g.

Therefore, weight of 20 drops of liquid = $(y_1 - x_1)$ g

Weight of 1 drop of liquid = $\dfrac{y_1 - x_1}{20} = w_1$ g

Similarly, the weight of 1 drop of water = $\dfrac{y_2 - x_1}{20} = w_2$ g

Then, $\gamma_1 = \dfrac{w_1}{w_2} \cdot \gamma_2$ where γ_2 is the surface tension of water which is taken as 72 mN/m.

Report : The surface tension of the liquid (glycerin) is _________ mN/m at _________ °C.

Notes : ST of few common liquids at 20 °C in mN/m

Water	72
Glycerin	63.4
Liquid paraffin	33.1
Benzene	35.0

Questions and Answers

1. What is interfacial tension? Is it different from ST?

    Ans : Generally speaking a boundary with a gas is known as surface and other boundaries being referred as interfaces. Accordingly the term ST is used when tension of liquid is measured in a liquid – gas system and interfacial tension refers to the tension at the interface of liquid–liquid or liquid–solid system.

    Actually every surface is an interface and thus there is no difference between surface and interface. Similarly ST and Interfacial tension are same, they are not different. But the tension between the phases needs to be mentioned.

2. What are the other methods of determination of ST?

   Ans :

   - Drop count method using stalagmometer.
   - Capillary rise method.
   - Du Nouy Ring Tensiometric method etc.

3. How is interfacial tension between two liquids determined?

   Ans : Refer next experiment where ST determination by drop count method is discussed.

4. What is the effect of temperature on ST?

   Ans : ST of liquids decrease with rise in temperature, if molecular composition remains same.

   In calculation of ST of liquid, the ST of the reference liquid at the temperature of experiment is used.

5. What are the importances of ST /Interfacial Tension in Pharmacy?

   Ans :

   - Interfacial tension between two immiscible liquids phases is critical in emulsion formulation. The emulsifying agent reduces their tension and helps in emulsification.
   - Reduction in interfacial tension and through formation of micelle by use of solubilizing agents improves solubilization of poorly water-soluble drugs. Aqueous preparation of oily vitamins is an example. Solubilized products are better absorped.
   - Reduction in interfacial tension between solid and water helps in improving contact and thus wetting. Improving wetting of hydrophobic drugs improves dissolution and absorption. Wetting of a solid in water is a prerequisite for suspension formulation.

9.2.2 Determination of Surface Tension by Drop Count Method

Aim : To determine the surface tension of a liquid (glycerin) by drop counting method using stalagmometer.

Principle :

The ratio of the weight of a drop of the liquid (w_1) to that of a reference substance (w_2) falling from the same capillary orifice is equal to the ratio of their surface tensions.

If γ_1 and γ_2 are the surface tensions of liquid and the reference standard respectively, then $\dfrac{\gamma_1}{\gamma_2} = \dfrac{w_1}{w_2}$

The weight of single drop is equal to $v\rho/n$, where v is the volume of liquid delivered; n is number of drops; ρ is density.

Then the above equation becomes : $\dfrac{\gamma_1}{\gamma_2} = \dfrac{\dfrac{v\rho_1}{n_1}}{\dfrac{v\rho_2}{n_2}}$

If the same volume of liquid and reference substance is allowed to flow from the same stalagmometer, then $\dfrac{\gamma_1}{\gamma_2} = \dfrac{\rho_1}{\rho_2} \times \dfrac{n_2}{n_1}$ or, $\gamma_1 = \dfrac{\rho_1}{\rho_2} \times \dfrac{n_2}{n_1} \times \gamma_2$

From the above equation, it is clear that if the densities and the numbers of drops of both the liquids are known, the surface tension can be calculated.

Water is generally used as reference liquid.

Apparatus and materials required : Stalagmometer, glycerin, water, specific gravity bottle and balance.

Process :

(i)   The cleaned stalagmometer is fixed perpendicularly with a clamp & stand and then filled with water by sucking.

(ii) The flow rate of water is controlled at the rate of 10-15 drops per minute by keeping a clamped rubber tube or fingertip at the top.

(iii) The numbers of drops are counted as they fall when the meniscus passes between the mark C and D (fixed volume). The process is repeated to collect at least three readings.

(iv) The stalagmometer is then dried and experiment is repeated with the liquid whose ST is to be determined.

Observation and Calculation :   Room temperature : _________ °C.

Sl. No of Observation	Number of drops			
	Water (n_2)	Mean (n_2)	Liquid (n_1)	Mean (n_1)
1.				
2.				
3.				

Other data required are : Density of the liquid and water (the reference standard), which can be determined following the procedure, described under density determination experiments.

$$\gamma_1 = \frac{\rho_1}{\rho_2} \times \frac{n_2}{n_1} \times \gamma_2$$

Report : The surface tension of the liquid (glycerin) is _______ mN/m at _______ °C.

Questions and Answers

1. How can the interfacial tension between two immiscible liquids be determined?

   Ans : This can be measured by dropping the denser liquid into the lighter one. The drops that formed under the lighter liquid are larger than those forms in air due to buoyancy effect.

   Taking the example of benzene and water:

   Number of drops of water formed in air and the number of drops of water formed under benzene from the same volume and the same stalagmometer is to be observed.

   Then the interfacial tension between water and benzene is

   $$\gamma_{wb} = \frac{\rho_w - \rho_b}{\rho_w} \cdot \frac{n_{air}}{n_b} \cdot \gamma_w$$

   where γ_w = ST of water; n_{air} and n_b = number of drops of water formed in air and benzene respectively; ρ_w and ρ_b are the density of water and benzene respectively.

9.3   Determination of Critical Micelle Concentration (CMC)

Aim : To determine the critical micelle concentration (CMC) of a surfactant (Sodium lauryl sulphate) by surface tension measurement.

Principle : The surface-active agents (surfactants) concentrate at the surface of a solution or at the interface between two immiscible liquids or between a liquid and a solid. They reduce the surface tension or interfacial tension.

As the total concentration of surface active agents in aqueous phase is gradually increased, the concentration of surface active agents undergoing adsorption at the surface is increased and this results in gradual reduction of surface or interfacial tension. At one point both the surface and bulk of aqueous phase become saturated with monomers of the surface active agents. This concentration point is known as CMC. At this point the surface or interfacial tension is reduced to the lowest value. Further increase in concentration of surface active agent will result in aggregation of monomers forming micelle without any appreciable change in surface tension.

The surface tension Vs concentration curve for an aqueous solution of surfactant shows a progressive decrease in surface tension until the CMC is reached.

The CMC is taken at the point of interaction of the extrapolated straight lines on either side of the break in the curve.

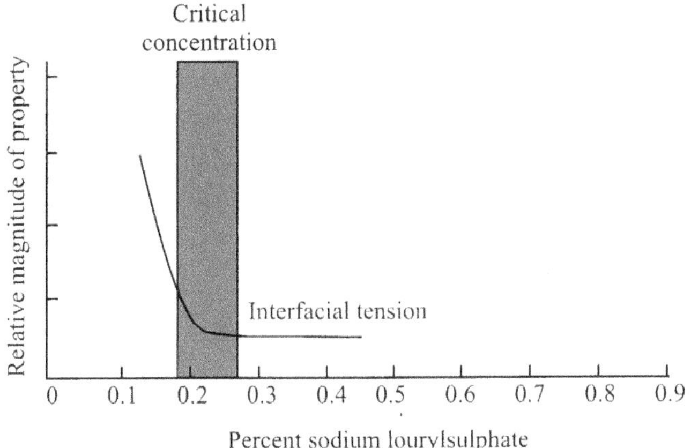

Apparatus and Materials required : Stalagmometer, Pycnomter, Sodium lauryl sulphate (SLS).

Process :

(i)   A stock solution of 5% sodium lauryl sulphate is prepared by dissolving 5 g of sodium lauryl sulphate in 100 ml water in a volumetric flask.

(ii)   A series of concentration of surfactant (SLS) is prepared by diluting the stock solution: 50 mg/100 ml (1 ml to 100 ml), 100 mg /100 ml (2 ml to 100 ml), 150 mg /100 ml (3 ml to 100 ml), 200 mg /100 ml (4 ml to 100 ml), 250 mg /100 ml (5 ml to 100 ml), 300 mg /100 ml (6 ml to 100 ml), 400 mg / 100 ml (8 ml to 100 ml) and 500 mg / 100 ml (10 ml to 100 ml).

(iii)   Surface tension of the prepared solutions is determined by drop count method.

(iv)   A graph of surface tension in Y-axis and concentration in X-axis is plotted.

(***Note :*** CMC: the concentration of monomers at which micelles form is termed as critical micelle concentration. The number of monomers that aggregate to form a micelle is known as "aggregate number" of the micelle. Normally the aggregate number is ≥ 50)

Observation and Calculation :   Room Temperature : _________ ºC.

Sample	Concentration in mg / 100ml	Number of drops (mean of three observations)	Density	Surface tension
Water	0			
I	50			
II	100			
III	150			
IV	200			
V	250			
VI	300			
VII	400			
VI	500			

The surface tension can be calculated for each concentration using the procedure described in experiment "Determination of surface tension by drop counting method".

CMC is determined from the surface tension Vs concentration curve.

Report : The CMC of SLS is ______mg/100 ml. (usually the concentration should be expressed in moles per litre. The concentration in mg/1000 ml should be divided by 1000 M where M is the molecular weight to get concentration in moles per litre.) (The approximate value of CMC of SLS is 180 – 260 mg / 100 ml)

Questions and Answers

1. What are the other methods of determination of CMC?

    Ans : Many other physical properties change at CMC i.e. conductivity, refractive index,, osmotic pressure and density. The measurement of these values help in determining the CMC.

    CMC can also be estimated by addition of traces of third component whose absorption spectrum depends on formation of micelle. A sharp change in slope of plot of Absorbance Vs concentration in log scale indicates the CMC value.

2. What are the importances of CMC in Pharmacy?

    Ans : Since solubilisation occurs above CMC value, this parameter helps in deciding the amount of surfactant required for solubilization. The solubilization has wide application:

- Preparation of aqueous products of poorly soluble drugs. Insoluble and soluble drugs can be formulated together. Water soluble and fat-soluble vitamins are formulated together (multivitamin liquids).

- Solubilized products have better bioavailability than suspensions and solid dosage forms. They have better appearance and taste too.

- Stability of some drugs increased if formulated in solubilized form. Vitamin A is more resistant to auto-oxidation in solubilized system than in oil.

10

Buffer

10.1 Preparation of Buffer

Aim : To prepare 100 ml of a pharmaceutical buffer of pH 5.0 (acetate buffer) and verify the same by measuring pH using a pH meter.

Principle : Buffers are compounds or mixtures of compounds; when present in solution, resist change of pH upon addition of small quantity of acid or alkali. Such solutions are called buffer solutions and are usually solutions of weak acids (or bases) and their corresponding salts (acetic acid and sodium acetate; ammonia and ammonium chloride).

The buffer equation is utilized to find out the quantity of weak acid and salt; or weak base and salt; required to get a buffer solution of desired pH. The buffer equation (also known as Henderson – Hasselbalch equation):

For weak acid and its salt:

$$pH = pK_a + \log\frac{[salt]}{[acid]}\;;\; \text{and for acetate buffer of pH 5.0, the equation is:}$$

$$5.0 = 4.76 + \log\frac{[salt]}{[acid]}, \text{ or, } \frac{[salt]}{[acid]} = \frac{1.74}{1}$$

The mole fraction of salt in the solution $= \dfrac{1.74}{1.74 + 1} = 0.635$

The concentration of salt in the buffer solution (mole fraction) = 63.5%

Concentration of acid in the buffer solution (mole fraction) = 36.5%

The quantity of acetic acid required $= \dfrac{36.5 \times \text{Mol.wt}}{1000} \times 100 \text{ g} = 219.18 \text{ g.}$

(the molecular weight of acetic acid is 60.05)

Then the weight of acetic acid is converted to volume using weight per ml data.

$$\text{The quantity of sodium acetate} = \frac{63.5 \times \text{Mol.wt}}{1000} \times 100 = 521.20 \text{ g.}$$

(the molecular weight of sodium acetate is 82.08)

Apparatus and materials required : Standard buffers, Acetic acid, Sodium acetate, and pH meter.

Process :

    (i)   The quantity of acetic acid and sodium acetate are dissolved in around 90 ml of distilled water and the volume is adjusted to 100 ml.

   (ii)   The pH meter is calibrated using standard buffer.

  (iii)   The pH of buffer solution is recorded.

Observation and Calculation :

Room temperature : _________ $^{\circ}$C

The pH of prepared buffer solution is _________.

Report : The prepared buffer solution has pH _________.

Questions and Answers

1. What is pH?

   Ans : pH is negative log of hydronium ion concentration ($pH = -\log [H^{+}]$). The pH scale ranges from 0-14, which indicates the acidity or alkalinity of a solution. pH 0-7 indicates acidity and 7-14 indicates alkalinity while pH 7.0 is neutral. Increase of pH indicates a decrease in acidity and increase in alkalinity.

2. What are standard buffers?

   Ans : These are buffer solutions that are used as indicators for particular pH. They are prepared from buffer tablets or weighing the individual ingredients (like potassium hydrogen phthalate) in distilled water. They are used to calibrate or validate pH meter.

3. What are the importances of buffers in pharmacy?

   Ans :

       (i)   Blood is maintained at a pH of around 7.4 by carbonic acid/ bicarbonate and acid/alkali sodium salt of phosphoric acid.

(ii) Tear's pH is also maintained at 7.4. Ophthalmic solutions are buffered to match with tear.

(iii) pH of pharmaceutical products are often determining factor for stability and physiological activity. Enzymes have maximum activity and stability at definite pH.

Ex: Pepsin has maximum activity at pH 1.5 and is effective in gastric fluid while it becomes inactive in duodenum where pH is around 8.

The vitamins are often stable only on narrow pH range. The pH needs to be adjusted for such products.

4. How do you select the pair of acid and its salts for buffers?

Ans : A weak acid is to be selected having pK_a approximately equal to pH of the desired buffer.

5. Why weak bases and their salts are not preferred for making buffers?

Ans : Weak bases are not preferred because of their volatility and instability and dependence of their pH on pK_w, which is often affected by temperature change.

6. How do buffers resist change of pH on addition of acid or alkali?

Ans :

(i) When sodium hydroxide (NaOH) is added to a buffer of acetic acid and sodium acetate; it reacts with acetic acid.

Sodium hydroxide + acetic acid $\Leftrightarrow$ Sodium acetate

Sodium acetate is less alkaline compared sodium hydroxide and thus change of pH is less.

(ii) When hydrochloric acid is added to the same buffer: we have

Hydrochloric acid + Sodium acetate $\Leftrightarrow$ acetic acid

Acetic acid is less acidic than hydrochloric acid.

The buffers do not maintain pH at an absolute constant value; but changes in pH are relatively small when small amount of acid or base are added.

10.2   Determination of Buffer Capacity

Aim : To determine the buffer capacity of acetate buffer at various concentrations and find out the pH of maximum buffer capacity.

Principle : The magnitude of resistance of a buffer to pH changes is called buffer capacity (β). The buffer capacity is defined as the ratio of the increment of strong base (or acid) to small change in pH brought about by this addition

$\beta = \Delta B/\Delta pH$ where ΔB is the small increment in gram equivalent per litre of strong base added to the buffer solution to produce a pH change of ΔpH.

The buffer capacity is not a fixed value for a given buffer system, but depends on the amount of base added.

When sodium hydroxide is added to acetate buffer (acetic acid + sodium acetate), the concentration of sodium acetate, the salt term in buffer equation, increases and the acetic acid concentration decreases proportionately. The changes in concentration of the salt and the acid by addition of a base are represented in buffer equation as:

$$pH = pK_a + \log\frac{[\text{salt}] + [\text{base}]}{[\text{acid}] - [\text{base}]}$$

when sodium hydroxide is added to a solution of acetic acid (excess), a mixture of acetic acid and sodium acetate formed. If sodium hydroxide addition is continued, there will be change in pH of the mixture, and buffer capacity at each point can be determined from the equation described above.

A plot of buffer capacity Vs pH will identify the pH at which buffer capacity is maximum.

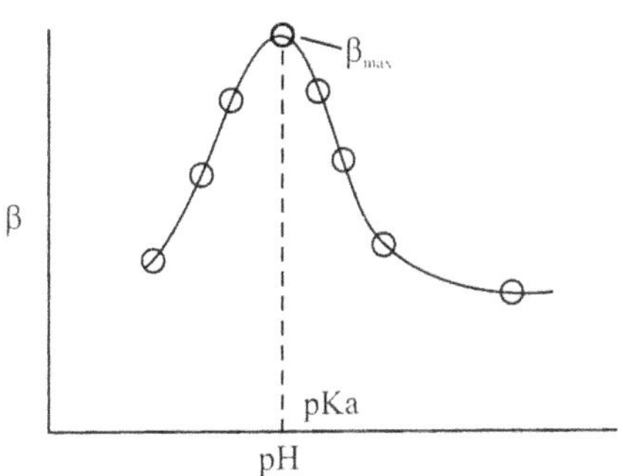

Apparatus and materials required : Standard buffers, 0.4 M Acetic acid, 0.2 M Sodium hydroxide, pH meter, burette, and pipettes.

Process :

    (i)   The pH meter is calibrated using standard buffer.

    (ii)   20 ml of 0.4 M acetic acid is taken in a beaker or conical flask and pH is recorded.

    (iii) 10 ml of 0.2 M sodium hydroxide is added to the acetic acid solution and pH of the mixture is recorded after through mixing. The process is repeated adding 2 ml 0.2 M sodium hydroxide every time till at least 30 ml sodium hydroxide is added.

    (iv)   Buffer capacity is calculated at each stage of addition.

Observation and Calculation :

20 ml of 0.4 M acetic acid solution is mixed with

ml of 0.2 M sodium hydroxide added	pH	Total volume of solution in ml	Difference in pH (ΔpH)	gram equivalent/ litre of base (ΔB)	$\beta = \dfrac{\Delta B}{\Delta pH}$
0			-------	--------	------
10					
12					
14					
16					
18					
20					
22					
24					
26					
28					
30					
24					

Calculation for moles of sodium hydroxide added :

1000 ml of one Molar sodium hydroxide solution = 1 mol of sodium hydroxide.

Therefore, 2 ml of 0.2 M sodium hydroxide solution = $\dfrac{1 \times 2 \times 0.2}{1000}$ mol of sodium hydroxide.

When x ml of 0.2 M sodium hydroxide is added to a volume of 20 ml 0.4 M acetic acid, the total volume is (20 + x) ml; thus the concentration is

$\dfrac{1 \times x \times 0.2}{1000 \times (20 + x)}$ mol/ml.

Thus, the molar concentration of sodium hydroxide after every 2 ml

addition $= \dfrac{1 \times x \times 0.2 \times 1000}{1000 \times (20 + x)} = \dfrac{x \times 0.2}{(20 + x)}$ moles per litre (M), where x is ml of 0.2 M sodium hydroxide added.

The pH at which the buffer capacity is maximum can be obtained from a plot of buffer capacity in Y-axis and pH in X-axis as shown in the graph:

Report :

(i)   The buffer capacity of acetate buffer:

Moles of sodium hydroxide added	Buffer capacity

(ii)   pH of maximum buffer capacity is ________ .

Questions and Answers

1. What is the unit of buffer capacity?

Ans : Mole (M) is the unit of buffer capacity.

2. What are the factors that influence buffer capacity?

Ans : The buffer capacity is not a fixed value of a buffer system. It depends on: (a) ratio of [Salt]/[Acid], the buffer capacity increases as the ratio approaches unity; (b) the magnitude of individual concentrations of the buffer components, the buffer becoming more efficient   as the salt and acid concentration increases.

Where [Salt]/[Acid] = 1, the buffer has maximum capacity.

3. pH is measured at each stage of alkali addition. Is there any other method by which pH can be determined at each point?

Ans : pH at each stage can be calculated from modified buffer equation:

$$pH = pK_a + \log \frac{[\text{salt}] + [\text{base}]}{[\text{acid}] - [\text{base}]}$$

4. What are the importances of buffer capacity?

Ans :

(i) It helps in preparing buffer of maximum usefulness. A buffer solution is normally useful within a range of $\pm$ 1pH unit of the pK_a of its acid. The acetate buffer is effective over a wider pH range, between 3.8 and 5.8 (i.e., when pH $=$ pK_a ±1).

(ii) The buffer capacity of blood is in the range of pH 7.0 to 7.8. The pH of blood is maintained by the primary buffers (carbonate – bicarbonate buffer and phosphate buffer) in plasma and secondary buffers (haemoglobin /oxyhaemoglobin and acid/ alkali potassium salts of phosphoric acid) in the erythrocytes. When the pH of blood goes below 6.9 or above 7.8, life is in serious danger.

(iii) *Importance in formulation :*

    (a) Lower buffer capacity solutions (ophthalmic products, injections) cause less irritation caused due to pH difference between solutions to be administered and the physiological environment. Low buffer capacity buffer boric acid solution causes less eye irritation than phosphoric acid buffer solution of same pH, when administered.

    (b) Injection solutions are usually not buffered. If they need to be buffered, the solutions should be buffered to a low capacity so that the buffers of blood may readily bring them within the physiologic pH range.

    (c) *Buffered Aspirin :* Aspirin is more rapidly absorbed from a system buffered at low buffer capacity than containing no buffer or highly buffered preparation. The buffer capacity of the buffer used in preparing buffered aspirin should be optimized to provide environment for rapid absorption with minimal gastric irritation, usually associated with aspirin.

11

Micromeritics

Micromeritics is the science and technology of small particles. It involves the study of particle size and size distribution, shape, angle of repose, porosity, true volume, bulk volume, true density and bulk density.

The unit of particle size is micrometer (μm) or simply micron (μ), which is equal to 10^{-6} meter or 10^{-3} millimetre. The millimicron (mμ) is referred as nanometer (nm).

The size and the surface area of particles have profound importance in pharmacy. Few important influence of particle size are mentioned below:

- Small particles will have large surface area leading to faster dissolution and drug absorption.
- Particle size and shape influence flowability of powders. The good flow property is an important requirement for tablet and capsule manufacturing.
- Particle size is important for proper mixing of granules and powders.
- The physical stability of suspension is dependent on size of dispersed particles. Smaller the particle the slower is the rate of settling (stokes' law).

In the present chapter, the experiments for particle size analysis and experiments involving derived properties of powders are discussed.

11.1 Calibration of Eye Piece Micrometer

Aim : To calibrate the eyepiece micrometer.

Principle : The eyepiece micrometer has 100 divisions. The determination of actual length of each division is known as calibration. The calibration is done in comparison with the standard stage micrometer. The number of divisions of eyepiece micrometer matching equally or coinciding with number of divisions of stage micrometer is the basis for calibration. Each division of stage micrometer is equal to 10 μm.

Materials and apparatus required : Microscope, eyepiece micrometer, standard stage micrometer.

Process :

    (i)   The eyepiece micrometer is matched with stage micrometer in such a way that the first line of both the micrometers coincide.

    (ii)   Then it is carefully looked to find out another point where lines of two micrometers coincide.

    (iii)   The number of divisions of eyepiece micrometer that equals to the number of divisions of stage micrometer is worked out.

Observation and Calculation :

Number of divisions of eyepiece micrometer (X) = Number of divisions of stage micrometer (Y);

$$\text{One division of eyepiece micrometer} = \frac{Y}{X} \text{ number of divisions of stage}$$

micrometer

As 1 division of stage micrometer is equal to 10 μm, the one division of

$$\text{eyepiece micrometer} = 10 \times \frac{Y}{X} \text{ μm.}$$

Report : One division of eyepiece micrometer = _______ μm

11.2   Determination of Particle Size and Size Distribution by Microscopy

Aim : To determine the average particle size of the given powder and study their size distribution by microscopy.

Principle : Determination of particle size as mean diameter is based on direct observation under microscope. Any collection of particles is usually polydisperse and it is necessary to know how many particles exist of what size. This is size range. Size range and the number of particles in each size are referred as size distribution.

In microscopy size of the particles needs to be measured in two directions (length and breadth). The microscope is fitted with calibrated eyepiece micrometer (or else, the eyepiece micrometer needs to be calibrated as discussed in previous experiment). At least 300-500 particles are to be measured to get a good estimation of distribution.

Materials and apparatus required : Microscope with eyepiece micrometer, glass slides, cover slip and powder sample.

Process :

(i)   The eyepiece micrometer is calibrated if not already calibrated.

(ii)   A suspension of the representative sample is prepared (preferably in liquid paraffin/turpentine oil) and little of it is mounted on a glass slide. The mounted material is placed on mechanical stage to observe through a microscope.

(iii) The particle diameter in both directions (length and breadth) is measured and recorded for at least 300 particles.

(iv)   The data is represented as size frequency distribution curve and average particle size is calculated.

Observation and Calculation :

Each division of eyepiece micrometer = _______ . _______ μm.

S. No.	Number of division (length)	Size (length) in μm	Number of division (breadth)	Size (breadth) in μm	Average size in μm
1.					
2.					
3.					
300					

Size range (μm)	Mean size range (μm) (X)	No. of particles (N) in each class interval	N.X
0 - 5	2.5		
5 - 10	7.5		
10 - 15	12.5		
15 - 20	17.5		
55 - 60	57.5		
		$\Sigma N =$	$\Sigma N.X =$

$$\text{Average particle size} = \frac{\sum N.X}{\sum N} \; \mu m$$

These data can be expressed in the form of bar graph or histogram. The mean of each class interval are connected to get distribution curve.

Report : The average particle size is found to be _______ mm. The distribution pattern is expressed in the figure.

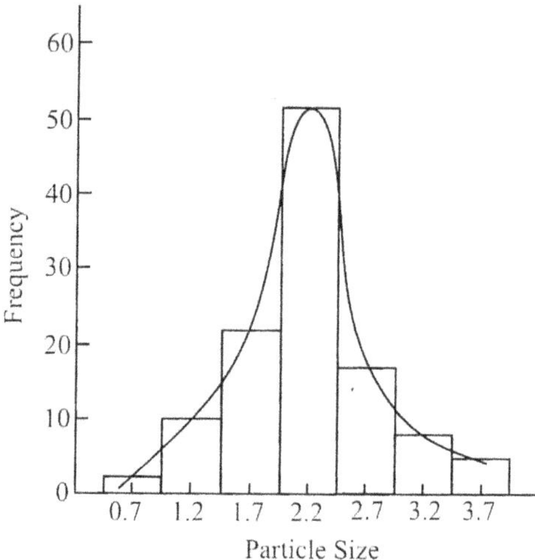

Questions and Answers

1. What are the advantages of optical microscopy in size determination?

   Ans : The advantage is relatively low cost of equipment with reasonably good accuracy. But it is a time consuming process, as large number of particles need to be counted to get reasonably good accuracy of distribution pattern.

2. What size range of particles can be measured by this method?

   Ans : 0.2 to 100 μm (approximately)

3. Is there any other way to express particle size distribution in a sample other than frequency curve and histogram?

   Ans : Yes, it can also be expressed as cumulative distribution curve.

   The percentage of particles can be calculated in each class interval and added cumulatively. Then the graphs are plotted as particle size Vs cumulative percentage less than stated size (under size) and particle size Vs over size.

Mean class interval in µm	Number of particles in each class interval	Percentage of particles	Cumulative percentage	
			Under size	Over size
2.5				
7.5				
12.5				
17.5				
-				
-				
-				
57.5				
	$\Sigma N =$			

Cumulative distribution curve

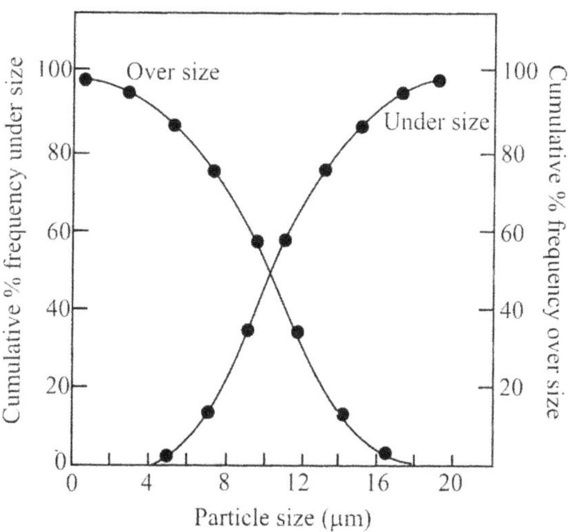

4. What are the other measurement parameters for expressing particle size measured by microscopy?

   Ans : Feret diameter, Martin diameter, Projected area diameter (Details are beyond the scope of this practical text. Interested readers can refer any standard text on physical pharmacy).

11.3   Determination of Particle Size and Size Distribution by Sieving

Aim : To determine the average particle size and find out their distribution pattern (by sieve analysis) of the supplied granular sample.

Principle : Sieve is a perforated screen and size of the opening depends on the number of meshes and the diameter of the wire constituting the mesh. The particles sufficiently small will pass through and those that are over size will be retained on the sieve. A sieve will classify the particles as less than the dimension of mesh (under size) and more than the dimension of mesh (over size).

When a powder sample is passed through a set of around 5 sieves arranged with descending aperture size (coarsest sieve at the top); the weight remaining on each sieve quantifies the over size particles. The particle size analysis through sieving is best expressed in the form of a cumulative over size, cumulative under size or as a histogram.

Unlike microscopy, in sieving the distribution is expressed on weight basis (weight diameter).

Materials and apparatus required : Granular sample, Series of sieves, Mechanical sieve shaker.

Method :

    (i)   About 5 sieves are arranged keeping one above the other in a series with the coarsest (less No) at the top and the finest at the bottom.

    (ii)   Around 100 gram of pre-weighed sample is placed on the top sieve.

    (iii)   The nest of sieves is shaken for about 20 minutes preferably in sieve shaker.

    (iv)   The quantity of sample retained on each sieve is weighed.

    (v)   The average particle size is determined as weight fraction and the distribution is expressed in a cumulative over size curve.

Observation and Calculation :

Sieve No. (Passed/ Retained)	Arithmetic mean of opening (mm)	Weight retained (g) in smaller sieve	% Retained	% Retained X Mean opening (mm)
20*/40	0.630			
40/60	0.335			
60/80	0.214			
80/100	0.163			
Total	---------		100.0	

* Assumed that no particle is retained in no. 20 sieve, all passed through.

$$\text{The average diameter} = \frac{\sum(\%\,\text{retained} \times \text{mean opening})}{100} = \text{---}\ \mu m.$$

The particle size weight distribution can best be expressed either as cumulative over size or cumulative under size.

Sieve number	Arithmetic mean of opening (mm)	Weight retained (g)	Cumulative % over size	Cumulative % under size
20	————	————	0.00	100
40				
60				
80				
100			100	

Report : The average diameter of the particles of the sample is ————— mm (Weight diameter). The distribution pattern is shown in the figure as cumulative over size and cumulative under size.

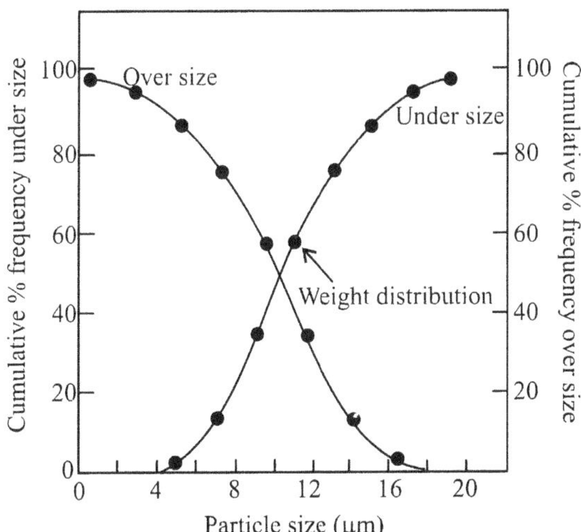

Questions and Answers

1. What size range of particles be usually analysed by sieving?

   Ans : Approximate size range of particles should be between 40 μm to 4700 μm.

2. What are the important factors that influence the particle size analysis by sieving method?

   Ans : Sieve loading, duration and intensity of shaking (agitation) influence the result. The particles shape too influences.

3. How do sieving differs from microscopy as a method for particle size analysis?

   Ans :

   - Approximate particle size range handles: Sieving: 40 µm to 4700 µm; Microscopy: 0.5 mm to 100 mm.
   - Sieving – Indirect measurement (size below or above the sieve size); Microscopy – Direct measurement.
   - Sieving – weight distribution; Microscopy – number distribution.

4. What are the utilities of sieve analysis?

   Ans : The average particle size (weight diameter) and their distribution can be determined especially of granules.

   The particles in a sample can be segregated depending on size.

11.4   Determination of Particle Size and Size Distribution by Andreasen Pipette

Aim : To determine the average particle size and study distribution pattern, using Andreasen Pipette, of the supplied powder sample (Zinc Oxide).

Principle : Particle size determination and distribution study using Andreasen Pipette utilizes the principle of sedimentation (stokes' law).

Stokes' law : Rate of settling $= \dfrac{h}{t} = \dfrac{d^2(\rho_s - \rho_l)g}{18\eta}$

Where d = diameter of the particle,

ρ_s = density of solid which is dispersed in the liquid,

ρ_l = density of the liquid in which the solid is dispersed,

g = acceleration due to gravity,

η = viscosity of the medium,

h = height of falling,

t = time of falling.

The diameter can be calculated by rearranging the stokes' equation:

$$d = \sqrt{\dfrac{18 h \eta}{(\rho_s - \rho_l) g t}}$$

Andreasen pipette is a vessel, as shown in the figure, consisting of 550 ml vessel containing a 20 ml pipette sealed into a ground glass stopper. The lower end of the pipette is 20 cm below the surface of the suspension from where sampling is done.

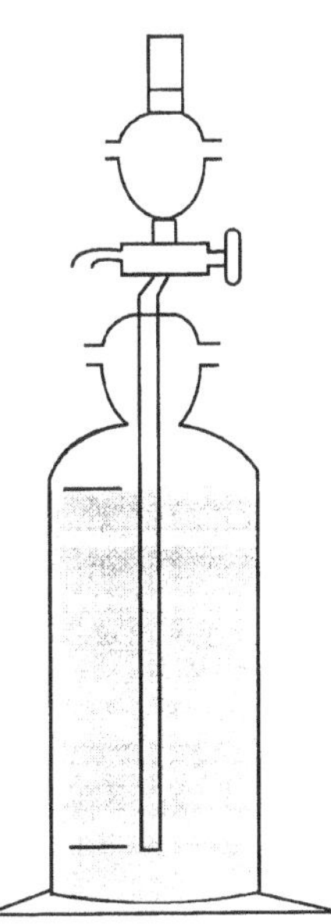

After addition of dispersion to the apparatus, withdrawal of samples at different intervals quantifies the amount of solids settled at that time interval. The quantity of powders present in each withdrawn sample can be determined through a suitable assay method. Gravimetry is preferred sometimes, as it does not involve any reagent. The weight of solid residue in each sample withdrawn is the weight fraction having particles of size less than the size obtained by the stokes' law calculation for that time period of settling. The weight of each sample residue is known as weight under size and the sum of successive weights is cumulative weight under size.

Materials and apparatus required : Andreasen pipette, weighing balance, sample (zinc oxide), liquid medium (water), deflocculating agent (sodium citrate)

Method :

    (i)   A suspension of 5.5 g zinc oxide in 50 ml water is prepared containing 2.75 g sodium citrate as deflocculating agent. The suspension is diluted to 550 ml with sufficient water to give a final concentration of 1%.

    (ii)   The suspension is introduced into the vessel up to 550 ml mark.

    (iii)   The vessel is stoppered and shaken to distribute the particles uniformly throughout the suspension.

    (iv)   The apparatus fitted with the pipette in place is clamped securely, preferably in a constant temperature bath.

    (v)   20 ml samples are withdrawn at predetermined time interval and discharged by means of two-way stopcock.

    (vi)   Samples are evaporated and weighed (correction for the quantity of flocculating agent is required).

Observation and Calculation :

The particle diameter corresponding to the various time periods is calculated from the stokes' law: The data are:

    Density of zinc oxide = 5.60 g/cc,

    Acceleration due to gravity = g = 981 cm/s^2,

Density of water = in g/cc (value can be determined or obtained referring appendix at room temperature; however, for practical purpose may be considered as 1 g/cc),

Viscosity of water = in g cm^{-1}.s^{-1} (value can be determined or obtained referring appendix at room temperature, however, for practical purpose may be considered as 1 cp i.e., 0.01g.cm^{-1}. s^{-1}),

Height = h = 20 cm.

Time in seconds (t)	Mean of class interval of corresponding spherical diameter in μm	Weight of sample collected (g) (under size)	Weight % of sample	Cumulative weight % under size
600				100.0
1200				
1800				
2400				
3000				
3600				
Total	----------		100.0	

The particle size distribution can be expressed as plot of *particle diameter* in X-axis and the *cumulative weight percent under size* in Y-axis.

The geometric mean diameter (the particle size at 50% probability level) can be calculated from the curve.

Report : The average particle size (particle size at 50% probability level) is ________ μm. The distribution pattern is shown in the figure as cumulative under size.

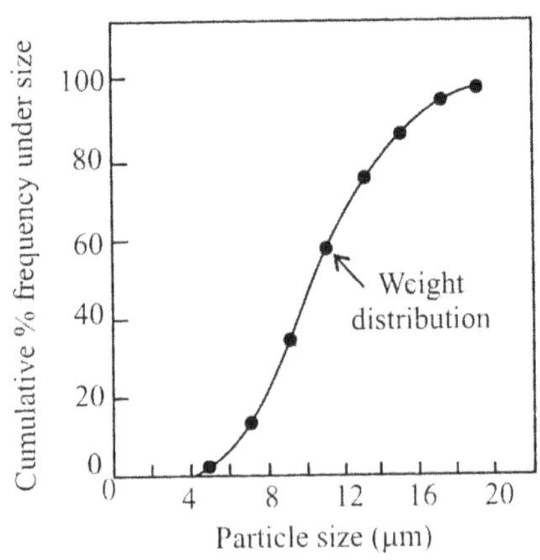

Questions and Answers

1. What range of particles be usually analysed by Andreasen apparatus?

   Ans : 2 to 200 μm.

2. What are the limitations of Andreasen pipette method?

   Ans :

   - Temperature control of settling medium is important because of possible change in density and viscosity with temperature.
   - The particle size range should be 2 to 200 μm.
   - Particle concentration should be between 1 to 2 %. Higher concentration may cause turbulent flow. Stokes' law is valid for laminar flow only.

3. What are other sedimentation methods of particle size measurement?

   Ans : There are two other methods: Micromerograph (powder particles settle in air) and Cahn sedimentation balance method (powders particles settle in a liquid). In these methods, the powder particles settle onto an ultra sensitive balance and weight is recorded cumulatively against time.

11.5   Determination of Specific Surface

Aim : To determine specific surface of Talc by adsorption method.

Principle : The specific surface is defined as surface area for unit weight or per unit volume. When a dissolved solid is adsorbed onto an adsorbent as monolayer, the surface area of the solid is equal to the surface area of adsorbent.

If surface area of the adsorbed solid is determined, then surface area of adsorbent and specific surface can be calculated. However, the surface area of one molecule of adsorbed solid must be known.

Stearic acid being a linear molecule, it gets adsorbed onto adsorbent as monolayer. The stearic acid adsorption on talc can be used in this experiment to find out the specific surface of talc.

Materials and apparatus required : Talc, stearic acid, conical flasks, burettes, pipettes, N/10 Na OH and phenolphthalein.

Procedure :

(i)   100 ml of 1.0% stearic acid solution is prepared in neutralized methanol (methanol is slightly acidic and is neutralized with dilute alkai).

(ii)   Around 5 g of talc is accurately weighed and taken in a stoppered conical flask.

(iii)   50 ml of 1.0% stearic acid in neutralized methanol is added to the conical flask containing talc.

(iv)   The mixture is thoroughly shaken from time to time for about 1 hr (The time required to attain adsorption equilibrium). The mixture is then left undisturbed for around 5 minutes.

(v)   The mixture is filtered through dry filters into a dry container (conical flask).

(vi)   10 ml of the filtrate (containing unadsorbed stearic acid) is pipetted out with a bulb pipette and titrated against N/10 Na OH solution using phenolphthalein as indicator.

(vii)   A blank titration is also performed using original 10 ml of 1.0 % stearic acid solution.

Observation and Calculation :

Room Temperature: _______ °C.

Weight of talc taken = _______ g (Let it be m g).

Titration with N/10 Na OH.

S. No.	Volume of N/10 Na OH in ml for 10 ml filtrate	Mean value of Volume of N/10 Na OH in ml	Concentration of stearic acid in Normality	Volume of N/10 Na OH in ml for 10 ml blank	Mean value of Volume of N/10 Na OH in ml	Concentration of stearic acid in original solution in Normality
1.						
2.						
3.						

If the Normality of original stearic acid solution = N_1 and Normality of filtrate (Equilibrium Normality) = N_2,

Then $(N_1 - N_2)$ equivalent / litre stearic acid is adsorbed.

As only 50 ml of stearic acid solution used, the quantity of stearic acid adsorbed

$$= \frac{(N_1 - N_2) \times \text{Equivalent weight of stearic acid} \times 50}{1000} \text{ g (Let it be x g)}$$

(Equivalent weight of stearic acid = Mol. wt of stearic acid = 284)

Now, m g of talc adsorbed x g stearic acid.

The surface area of m g talc   = Surface area of x g stearic acid.

No. of molecules in x g of stearic acid = $\dfrac{6.023 \times 10^{23}}{284} \times x$

[As 1 g molecule of any substance contains 6.023×10^{23} molecules; Avogadro's No.]

1 molecule of stearic acid has an area of 20.46×10^{-16} sq. cm.

Thus, $\dfrac{6.023 \times 10^{23}}{284} \times x$ g of stearic acid will have an area of

$$\dfrac{20.46 \times 10^{-16} \times 6.023 \times 10^{23}}{284} \times x \text{ sq. cm}$$

The surface area of m g of talc $\dfrac{20.46 \times 10^{-16} \times 6.023 \times 10^{23}}{284} \times x$ sq.

cm

$\therefore$ The   surface   area   of   1g   talc   would   be

$$\dfrac{20.46 \times 10^{-16} \times 6.023 \times 10^{23}}{284 \times m} \times x \text{ sq. cm.}$$

[The quantity of stearic acid adsorbed can simply be calculated from the relation:

1 ml of N/10 Na OH $\equiv$ 0.0284 g of stearic acid.

Quantity of stearic acid adsorbed per 10 ml of the mixture

= (Vol. of N/10 Na OH for blank - Vol. of N/10 Na OH for filtrate) $\times$ 0.0284 g]

Report : The specific surface of talc is _______ sq. cm. /g.

Questions and Answers

1. What are the other principles/methods used for determining specific surface?

 Ans :

 (i) Particle size and their distribution help in finding out surface area. For spherical particles, the surface area = πd^2 and specific surface = $6/\rho d$ where d = diameter and ρ = density.

 As the particles are generally not uniform and spherical, d_{vs} (volume - surface diameter) is used for calculating specific surface.

(ii) By using principle of adsorption of Nitrogen over the adsorbent.

(iii) By use of air permeability method that depends on the principle that rate at which gas or liquid permeates a bed of powder is related to the surface area exposed.

2. What is the significance of specific surface or surface area in pharmacy?

Ans :

(i) Surface area is related to dissolution. Larger the surface area quicker is the rate of dissolution, which indicates quicker absorption.

(ii) Larger surface area indicates better or more adsorption. Adsorption has several applications discussed in previous experiment.

3. Is there any other method to determine adsorbed amount by the adosrbent?

Ans : Yes. By using different concentration of stearic acid and performing the experiment as described under Freundlich adsorption isotherm constant experiment and plotting a curve using Langmuir's adsorption isotherm: $\dfrac{C}{x/m}$ Vs C; the value of constant b can be determined from the slope. (b is the amount of stearic acid required to produce an adsorbed mono layer over m g of talc).

12

Viscosity

12.1   Determination of Viscosity

Aim : To determine the viscosity of benzene using Ostwald's U tube viscometer.

Principle : The viscosity of a fluid is the internal resistance to flow. This is also called as coefficient of dynamic viscosity.

The relationship between the flow rate of a liquid through a capillary tube and the viscosity is the principle behind the determination of Newtonian fluids (fluids exhibiting stream line flow). This relationship is expressed in Poiseuille's equation :

$$V = \frac{P\pi r^4 t}{8l.\eta} \quad \text{or,} \quad \eta = \frac{P\pi r^4 t}{8l\,V}$$

Where V = Volume of liquid (cc) flowing in time t (second).

P = Driving pressure (dyne /cm^2).

r = Radius of the capillary (cm).

l = Length of the capillary (cm).

η = Coefficient of viscosity (poise).

When the P is due to force of gravity, then $P = h\,\rho\,g$, where h is height of liquid, ρ is the density of liquid and g is acceleration due to gravity.

Now, $\eta = \dfrac{h\rho g\pi r^4 t}{8l.\,V}$

When equal volume of two liquids (one test and the other reference standard whose viscosity is known) are flown through the same apparatus under same driving pressure, then

$$\frac{\eta_{test}}{\eta_{standard}} = \frac{P_{test} \cdot t_{test}}{P_{standard} \cdot t_{standard}}$$ as other terms: h, g, π, r, l and V

are equal for both test and standard and gets cancelled.

As absolute viscosity determination is difficult, the viscosity of a liquid can be determined easily by comparing with a liquid whose viscosity is known using the above equation

written as : $\eta_{test} = \eta_{standard} \cdot \dfrac{P_{test} \cdot t_{test}}{P_{standard} \cdot t_{standard}}$ and water can

be used as reference liquid whose viscosity is known.

The Ostwald's U tube viscometer is used for the determination of viscosity of Newtonian fluids.

Materials and apparatus required : Ostwald's U tube viscometer, pipette, stopwatch, density measurement facility, benzene and water.

Procedure :

(i)   The cleaned viscometer is vertically clamped.

(ii) Sufficient liquid whose viscosity is to be determined is poured using a pipette into bulb Y to reach the mark E.

(iii) The liquid is then sucked or blown up to a point 1 cm above A.

(iv) The time for the liquid to fall from A to B is measured using a stopwatch. This is repeated for three times to ensure that accurate time is only recorded.

(v)   The density of the liquid is measured using specific gravity bottle.

(vi) In the similar way, the data for the standard liquid (water) is recorded using the same apparatus after cleaning and drying.

Ostwald's viscometer

Observation and Calculation : Room Temperature : _________ °C.

Time for the liquid to fall from A to B (t $_{test}$) = _________ seconds.

Density of the liquid (determined separately) (r$_{test}$) = _________ g/cc.

Time for water to fall from A to B (t $_{standard}$) = _________ seconds.

Density of water (determined separately/can be obtained from appendix at room temperature) $(r_{standard}) =$ _______ g/cc.

$$\text{The viscosity of the liquid} = \eta_{test} = \eta_{standard} \cdot \frac{\rho_{test} \cdot t_{test}}{\rho_{standard} \cdot t_{standard}}$$

The viscosity of water at room temperature can be obtained from standard table (refer appendix).

The unit of viscosity as calculated in poise can be converted to SI units by multiplying the value with 10^{-1}.

Report : The viscosity of the liquid (benzene) at room temperature (specify) is _______ Pa.s. (the usual value is 5.6 mPa.s)

Viscosities of some liquids at 20 °C

Liquid	Viscosity in mPa.s (centipoises)
Benzene	5.6 at 30 °C
Chloroform	0.58
Castor oil	986
Ethanol	1.20
Glycerol	1490
Water	1.002

Questions and Answers

1. Can you measure the viscosity of all liquids using Ostwald's U tube viscometer?

   Ans : No. Normally the Newtonian fluids' viscosity can be measured by this viscometer. However, the measurement of viscosity of very viscous liquids in this apparatus is not convenient due to difficulty in filling and long time for falling. The suspended level viscometer can be used in such situations.

   For other liquids, Brookfield viscometer can be used.

2. How does temperature influence viscosity?

   Ans : The viscosity of liquid deceases with increase in temperature. As a rough guide, the viscosity of many liquids decreases by 2% for each degree rise in temperature.

   In case of gas, the increase in temperature causes increase in viscosity.

3. What is kinematic viscosity?

   Ans : When the coefficient of dynamic viscosity (viscosity) is divided by the density of the liquid, then it is called kinematic viscosity. The unit of this kinematic viscosity is stoke (corresponding viscosity unit is poise).

   The liquids of equal kinematic viscosity will flow at identical rates through a given tube, when the pressure causing the flow is due solely to the hydrostatic head of the liquid.

4. What are the importances of viscosity in pharmacy?

   Ans :

   (i) Viscosity is an important consideration for consistency or feel of a product and stability of suspensions. The rate of settling of insoluble solids in suspension is inversely proportional to viscosity (stoke's law).

   (ii) The viscosity of the injection should not be too high that it prevents the passage through the needle when the plunger is pushed.

   (iii) The viscosity of the gel is an important criterion for application. It needs to be pourable on shaking.

   (iv) Ophthalmic preparations are sometimes adjusted to certain viscosity so that they could not be easily washed off and thus to prolong the contact period.

   (v) By increasing viscosity, the stability of suspensions and emulsions can be improved.

13

Adsorption Isotherm

13.1 Determination of Freundlich Adsorption Isotherm Constant

Aim : To determine the constants of *Freundlich* adsorption isotherm for adsorption of acetic acid on charcoal.

Principle : The phenomena of accumulation of solids, dissolved in liquids, at the surface of another solid are known as adsorption (more generally at the interface of two phases). The gases too adsorb to solid surfaces in similar way. The adsorbate (that gets adsorbed) is adsorbed on the adsorbent (that adsorbs).

The extent of adsorption depends on the temperature. It deceases with increase of temperature where adsorption is an exothermic process. At a given temperature, the amount of adsorption increases with increase in concentration of adsorbate (when dissolved in liquid) or pressure (when in gas phase). *Freundlich* adsorption isotherm represents the variation in extent of adsorption with the equilibrium pressure or concentration of adsorbate at a fixed temperature.

The Freundlich adsorption isotherm for adsorption of a solid from a solution is conveniently expressed as:

$$\log \frac{x}{m} = \log k + \frac{1}{n} \log C \; ;$$

where x = Amount of adsorbate adsorbed by m g of adsorbent,

C = Equilibrium concentration of adsorbate,

k and n = Empirical constants.

The plot of $\log \dfrac{x}{m}$ (Y-axis) and log C (X-axis) makes a linear line with slope = 1/n and Y intercept = log k.

The value of k can be directly read from Y intercept from a plot on log - log paper.

When charcoal is added to a solution of acetic acid, the acetic acid gets adsorbed on charcoal. On filtration, the filtrate will contain the acetic acid, which can be determined titrimetrically. If free acetic acid were subtracted from the known total amount of acetic acid, it would give quantity of acetic acid adsorbed.

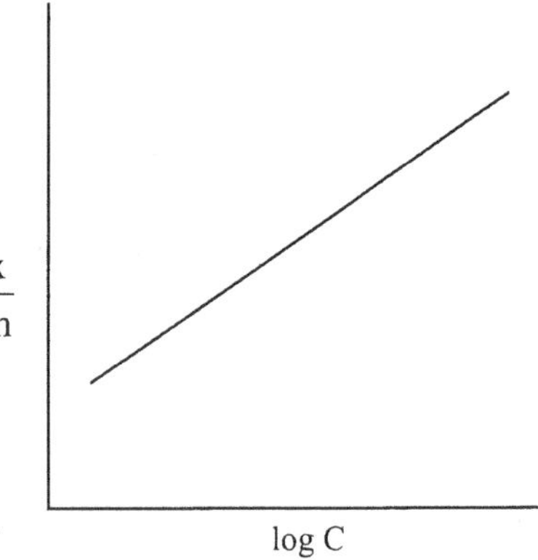

Apparatus and materials required :
Activated charcoal, N/2 acetic acid, N/10 sodium hydroxide, burette, pipettes, reagent bottles.

Process :

(i)   Around 2 g of powdered activated charcoal is accurately weighed and placed into each of cleaned and dried bottles numbered 1 to 5.

(ii)   Using burette 50, 30, 20, 10 and 5 ml quantities of N/2 acetic acid are added into the bottle numbers 1, 2, 3, 4 and 5 respectively. Similarly 0, 20, 30, 40 and 45 ml quantities of water are added to the bottle numbers 1 to 5 respectively (to make volume equal in all bottles).

(iii)   The bottles containing charcoal, acetic acid and water are vigorously shaken from time to time for about 30 minutes. The solution is then kept undisturbed for about 5 minutes.

(iv)   The solutions of each bottle are then filtered through dry filter papers and the filtrates are collected in properly labelled flasks, rejecting first 5-10 ml of filtrate in each case.

(v)   10 ml of these filtrates are pipetted out into different conical flasks and titrated against N/10 sodium hydroxide using phenolphthalein as indicator.

(vi)   10 ml of stock N/2 acetic acid is also titrated separately using N/10 sodium hydroxide.

Observation and calculation :

Room temperature: ________ °C.

10 ml of stock N/2 acetic acid solution = x ml of N/10 sodium hydroxide

Flask	Amount of charcoal in g (m)	Initial concentration of acetic acid before adsorption	Equilibrium concentration after adsorption (concentration in filtrate) (C)	Amount of acid adsorbed (x)	x/m	Log x/m	Log C
1		0.5 M					
2		0.3 M					
3		0.2 M					
4		0.1 M					
5		0.05 M					

Concentration of acetic acid in filtrate can be determined from this relation:

1000 ml N sodium hydroxide $\equiv$ 1000 ml N acetic acid

(normality and molarity value of acetic acid is same)

Amount of acid adsorbed (x) =

$$\frac{(\text{Initial concentration} - \text{Equlibrium concentration}) \times \text{Volume of acetic acid solution} \times \text{Mol. Wt.}}{1000} \, g$$

The volume in this experiment is 50 ml.

(Determination of slope is described separately in the appendix)

Slope = 1/n and the value of n can be calculated. And the k value can be determined from intercept log k.

Report : The value of n and k of acetic acid adsorption on charcoal adsorption isotherm is ______ and ______ .

Questions and Answers

1. What are the units of n and k of *freundlich* adsorption isotherm?

   Ans : n has no unit.

   $$\text{Unit of k is } \frac{\text{unit of amount of adsorbate adsobed}}{\text{unit of amount of adsobent}} \text{ ; in the present}$$

   experiment it is g /g.

2. What are the importance of n and k of Freundlich adsorption isotherm?

   Ans : In a given system, these constants are useful in determining the quantity of solute from solution adsorbed per unit weight of adsorbent, if equilibrium concentration is known.

3. How can the constants of Langmuir's adsorption isotherm be determined?

   Ans : Langmuir's adsorption isotherm equation expresses a quantitative relationship between the extent of adsorption and the equilibrium pressure or concentration. For adsorption of solutes from solution, the expression is:

   $$\frac{C}{x/m} = \frac{1}{ab} + \frac{1}{b}C$$

Where   C = equilibrium concentration of adsorbate,

        x = amount adsorbed by m g of adsorbent,

a and b are constants. a is the ratio of rate constants for adsorption and desorption process. b is the amount of adsorbate required to produce an adsorbed monolayer over the whole surface of adsorbent.

The experiments can be performed as described in the above experiment and a and b can be calculated from the plot of $\dfrac{C}{x/m}$ in Y-axis and C in X-axis. The slope is 1/b and intercept in Y-axis is 1/ab. The constant b is dimension less and has no unit while a has unit: $(conc.)^{-1}$.

4. What is the difference between Freundlich adsorption isotherm and Langmuir's adsorption isotherm?

   Ans : For solution: Freundlich adsorption isotherm explains the relationship between the extent of adsorption and concentration of adsorbate in solution at a fixed temperature (valid at low concentration), while Langmuir's adsorption isotherm explains the relationship between the extent of adsorption and equilibrium concentration of adsorbate, when monolayer is complete. In Langmuir's adsorption isotherm the rate of adsorption at any instant is proportional to the amount of free surface available at that instant.

5. What are the applications of adsorption principle and adsorbents in pharmacy?

   Ans :

   (i)   Used in the determination of surface area (discussed in next experiment).

   (ii) They are used as decolorizing agents. Ex: Activated charcoal.

   (iii) They are used as desiccating agents. The small pack of silica gel is sometimes included inside the container to protect the product from adverse effects of high humidity.

   (iv) It is a principle in adsorption chromatography.

   (v)   Charcoal and Kaoline have long been used as adsorbent for removal of toxic materials like poisons (atropine, strychnine etc.) from gastrointestinal tract.

14

Physical Stability of Suspension

Aim : To prepare a flocculated and deflocculated suspension of magnesium carbonate and assess their stability.

Principle : Magnesium carbonate is an insoluble but diffusible solid.

In flocculated suspension, the particles settle more quickly than particles of deflocculated one. But the sediments form a cake like structure in deflocculated suspension making dispersibility on shaking a big problem. Comparing these two types of suspensions, the flocculated one is pharmaceutically acceptable or preferable. However, a controlled flocculation is desirable to achieve controlled sedimentation with ease of dispersibility.

Electrolytes and ionic surfactants can be used as flocculating agents to produce a flocculated suspension. Suspension prepared without flocculating agents (drug and the solvent) is a deflocculated one.

The physical stability of the suspension is assessed by determining the sedimentation volume and/or degree of flocculation.

The suspensions can be prepared by using the formulae:

Flocculated Suspension		Deflocculated Suspension	
Magnesium carbonate	5 g.	Magnesium carbonate	5 g.
Aluminium chloride	0.1 g.		
Water to	100 ml.	Water to	100 ml.

Materials and apparatus required : Magnesium carbonate, aluminium chloride, water, pastle and mortar, measuring cylinders.

Procedure :

I.   Step : Preparation of Suspension

Deflocculated Suspension

(i)   The light magnesium carbonate is powdered in a mortar.

(ii) The water is added with trituration to make a cream and diluted sufficiently.

(iii) Then it is transferred to a measuring cylinder. The mortar is repeatedly rinsed with little water every time and the rinsed mixture is added subsequently to adjust the volume.

Flocculated Suspension

(i)   The light magnesium carbonate is powdered in mortar.

(ii) Aluminium chloride is dissolved in little water and added with trituration to make a cream. The cream is transferred to the measuring cylinder after dilution with water.

(iii) The mortar is repeatedly rinsed with little water every time and the rinsed mixture is added subsequently to adjust the volume.

II.   Step : Evaluation of Suspension

(i)   The suspensions in the cylinders are thoroughly shaken to make the dispersions uniform.

(ii) The cylinders are kept undisturbed on a flat surface after shaking.

(iii) The volume of sediment at different time: 0, 10, 30, 45 and 60 minutes is measured.

(iv) The sedimentation volume and degree of flocculation is calculated.

Observation and Calculation :

Original volume of suspension = 100 ml.

Time in minute	Flocculated Suspension		Deflocculated Suspension	
	Volume of sediment in ml (Vu)	Sedimentation volume (Vu/Vo)	Volume of sediment in ml (Vu)	Sedimentation volume (Vu/Vo)
0				
10				
30				
45				
60				

The degree of flocculation at one hour

$$= \frac{\text{sediment volume of flocculated suspension at 1 hour}}{\text{sediment volume of deflocculated suspension at 1 hour}}$$

(Though degree of flocculation is related to the ultimate sediment volume in flocculated and deflocculated suspension, it is not feasible to achieve or determine ultimate volume within the practical period. Hence the value at 1 hour is determined.)

The plot of sedimentation volume in Y-axis and time in X-axis is drawn.

Report : The flocculated and deflocculated suspensions are prepared and evaluated for sedimentation volume.

(Sedimentation volume quickly decreases in flocculated suspension compared to deflocculated suspension initially but ultimate sedimentation volume of flocculated suspension will be higher).

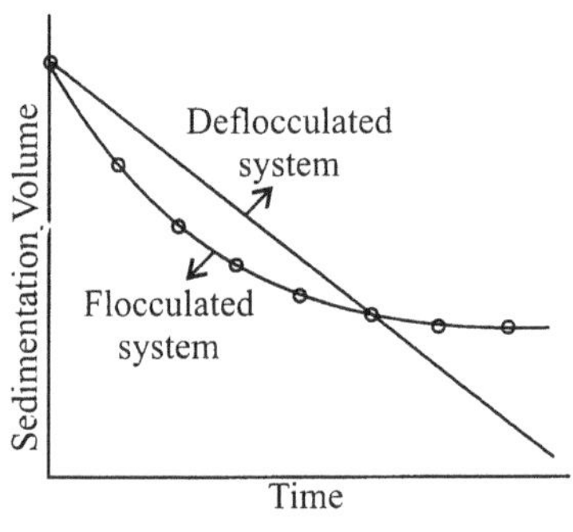

Note : In formulation development, several suspensions with different formula can be prepared and evaluated based on sedimentation volume to find out the best one. An assessment of slope of each line gives the indication which suspension shows the lowest rate of sedimentation. The more horizontal the curve is, the better is the suspension.

Questions and Answers

1. What are the differences between flocculated and deflocculated suspensions?

Ans :

Parameter	Flocculated Suspension	Deflocculated Suspension
Rate of settling	Fast	Slow
Sediment volume	High	Low
Redispersibility	Easy	Difficult

2. What are the parameters usually evaluated to assess the physical stability of suspensions?

   Ans : (i) Particle size, (ii) Sedimentation height or volume, (iii) Degree of flocculation (flocculation ratio), (iv) viscosity (v) Zeta potential

3. How do the above factors related to suspension stability?

   $$Ans : \text{Stoke's Law } v = \frac{D^2(\rho_s - \rho_l)g}{18\eta}$$

   where v = rate of settling,

   D = particle size (diameter),

   ρ_s and ρ_l are density of solid and dispersion medium. η = viscosity and g = acceleration due to gravity.

Parameter	Influence
Particle size	Rate of settling
Viscosity	Rate of settling
Degree of flocculation	Formulation of porous sediment and dispersibility
Sedimentation volume	Rate of settling
Zeta potential	Flocculated suspensions would have zeta potential close to zero. Controlled Flocculated Suspension is ideal for pharmaceutical suspensions. High zeta potential (negative or positive) confers stability. Moderate stability when zeta potential is between ± 30 and ± 60 mv; Good stability when it is ± 60 and ± 100 mv;

4. What are the units of sedimentation volume and degree of flocculation?

   Ans : They are ratio terms and hence have no units.

15

Physical Stability of Emulsion

Aim : To assess the physical stability of benzyl benzoate lotion (an emulsion for external use).

Principle : The physical stability of the emulsion is important to keep the dispersion intact. A stable emulsion is one in which the dispersed globules retain their initial character and remain uniformly distributed throughout the continuous phase. The unstable conditions in emulsions are: creaming, coalescence, cracking or breaking and phase inversion.

The physical stability of an emulsion can be assessed by an examination of the degree of creaming or coalescence occurring over a period of time. The ratio of volume of creamed part of an emulsion to the total volume is the required indicator. The globule size analysis can also be used to assess stability.

Materials and apparatus required : Benzyl benzoate, triethanol amine, oleic acid, water, beaker/conical flask, bottle.

Procedure :

1. **Preparation of emulsion (benzyl benzoate lotion)**

   (At least 3 emulsions are to be prepared using the same formula and in the laboratory, data from other students can be used)

   Formula for benzyl benzoate lotion :

Benzyl benzoate	25 ml.
Triethanol amine	0.5 g.
Oleic acid	2 g.
Water	75 ml.

   To make around 100 ml.

(The density of triethanol amine is 1.12 g/ml and that of oleic acid is 0.895 g/ml. This can be used to convert weight into volume)

(i)   Triethanol amine is mixed with oleic acid. Benzyl benzoate is added and mixed.

(ii)   The mixture is transferred to a bottle of around 200 ml capacity (double the volume required to prepare).

(iii)   25 ml water is added and the mixture is thoroughly shaken.

(iv)   The remaining 50 ml water is added and shaken thoroughly.

2.   Extent of creaming :

(i)   The prepared emulsion is transferred to a 100 ml measuring cylinder.

(ii)   The emulsion is left undisturbed in the cylinder and the volume of cream developed is noted over time from 0 to 2 hours at a frequency of every 30 minutes (as normal period of practical class is around 3 hrs).

(iii)   The graph is plotted taking degree of creaming in Y-axis and time in X-axis.

Observation and Calculation :

Number of observation	Time in minutes	Volume of cream in ml	Degree of creaming (Volume of cream ÷ Total volume of emulsion)
1.	0		
2.	30		
3.	60		
4.	90		
5.	120		

Report : The creaming instability of emulsions is observed in the following order: ________ > ________ > ________ .

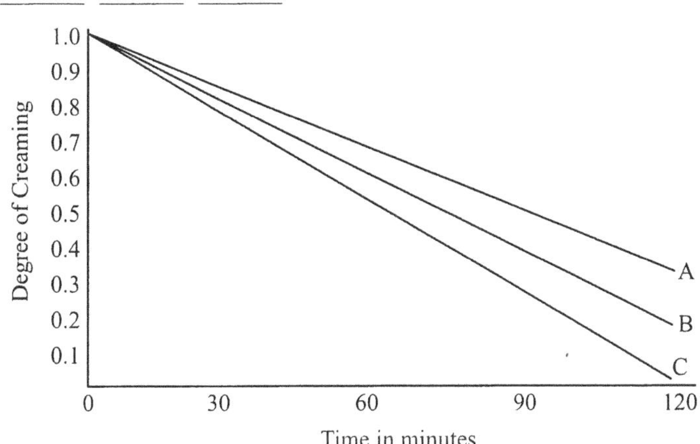

Questions and Answers

1. What is creaming?

   Ans : Creaming is the separation of an emulsion into two regions, one of which is richer in disperse phase than the other i.e., formation of concentrated emulsion either at bottom or top. The term is coined from the creaming of milk. The creaming occurs at the top for this emulsion (o/w).

2. What are the factors that influence creaming? How can this be reduced to stabilize emulsion?

   Ans : Stoke's law : $v = \dfrac{d^2\left(\rho_s - \rho_l\right)}{18\eta}g$

   where
   v = rate of settling,
   d = diameter of globules,
   ρ_s = density of globules (dispersed phase),
   ρ_l = density of dispersion medium,
   η = viscosity of the dispersion medium,
   g = acceleration due to gravity.

   The migration of globules of emulsion follows stoke's law. It thus depends on:

   (i) *Size of the globules :* Small size will have less creaming. Method of manufacture controls globule size and homogenisers can be used to reduce globule size.

   (ii) *Viscosity of the continuous phase :* Increase in viscosity (of course, without exceeding the limits of acceptable consistency) will reduce creaming and viscosity can be increased by adding agents like tragacanth, methyl cellulose and sodium alginate.

   (iii) *Density difference between the two phases :* Larger the density differences between internal phase and external phase, more will be creaming. Making the densities of two phases equal / identical will prevent creaming completely. But this is not practicable.

3. What are the reasons for cracking and how can that be avoided?

   Ans : Cracking or breaking of emulsion means complete separation of two phases. The adsorbed layer of the emulsifier around the globule, which stabilizes the emulsion, is destroyed. The internal phase globules tend to coalesce and cracking occurs.

Addition of common solvents, addition of emulsifiers of opposite charge, microbial contamination causing damage of interfacial film leads to cracking. Exposure to extreme temperature either high or low also leads to cracking.

Increasing viscosity of external phase increases stability. However, viscosity alone does not produce stable emulsion.

4. What are the differences of creaming and cracking?

Ans :

S.No.	Creaming	Cracking
1.	Aggregation of globules of internal phase at the top or bottom.	Coalescence of internal phase globules as separate layer.
2.	Reversible process.	Irreversible process.
3.	Simple shaking makes the emulsion usable.	Emulsion can not be reused.
4.	Inaccuracy of dosage if not properly shaken.	Emulsion can not be reused.

16

Complexation

16.1 Determination of Stability Constant of Complex

Aim : To determine the stability constant of glycine–copper complex by pH titration method.

Principle : Glycine and copper complex is a chelate type metal ion complex and the chelation of cupric ion by glycine is represented by:

$$Cu^{+2} + 2NH_3^+ CH_2COO^- = Cu(NH_2CH_2COO)_2 + 2H^+$$

In glycine copper complex, copper ion is the metal (M) and the glycine is the ligand (A).

The equation would be :

$$M + A = MA; \qquad K_1 = \frac{[MA]}{[M][A]}$$

$$MA + A = MA_2; \qquad K_2 = \frac{[MA_2]}{[MA][A]}$$

$$M + 2A = MA_2; \quad \text{and} \quad \beta = K_1K_2 = \frac{[MA_2]}{[MA][A]^2}$$

Where K_1 and K_2 are formation constants and β is the equilibrium constant for overall reaction (also known as stability constant).

The average number of ligand groups bound per metal ion is expressed as:

$$\bar{n} = \frac{[\text{Total Concentration of ligand bound}]}{[\text{Total Concentration of metal ion}]}$$

The concentration of free glycine [A] in this complexation reaction can be obtained as:

$$p[A] = \frac{1}{2}\log \beta \ \text{ at } \ \bar{n} = 1;$$

$$p[A] = \log K_1 \ \text{ at } \ \bar{n} = \frac{1}{2};$$

$$p[A] = \log K_2 \ \text{ at } \ \bar{n} = \frac{3}{2};$$

Apparatus and materials required : Glycine hydrochloride, cupric chloride, 0.259 N sodium hydroxide, pH meter, burette, beakers, volumetric flasks etc.

Process :

I.   **Titration of Glycine hydrochloride with Sodium hydroxide**

1. 100 ml glycine hydrochloride solution at 3.34×10^{-2} mole per litre concentration is prepared. (Molecular weight of glycine hydrochloride is 111.53. 0.372 g of glycine hydrochloride is required to be dissolved and volume is to be made 100 ml)

2. 75 ml glycine hydrochloride solution is pipetted out and taken in a conical flask. The pH of the solution is measured.

3. 0.259 N sodium hydroxide is added gradually and pH of the mixture is measured after each 1 ml addition of sodium hydroxide.

II.   **Titration of Glycine hydrochloride and Copper Complex with Sodium hydroxide**

1. 100 ml solution containing 3.34×10^{-2} mole per litre of glycine hydrochloride and 9.45×10^{-3} mole per litre of cupric chloride is prepared. (The molecular weight of cupric chloride is 134.45. 0. 127 g of cupric chloride is required).

2. 75 ml of glycine hydrochloride and cupric chloride solution is pipetted out and taken in a conical flask. The pH of the solution is measured.

3. 0.259 N sodium hydroxide is added gradually and pH of the mixture is measured after each 1 ml addition of sodium hydroxide.

III.   A graph is drawn taking volume of sodium hydroxide in X-axis and pH in Y-axis.

IV.   The value of $\bar{n}$ and p[A] at different pH are computed from the described equation.

V.   The formation curve is plotted using p[A] in X-axis and $\bar{n}$ in Y-axis.

VI. The value of $\log K_1$ at $\bar{n} = \dfrac{1}{2}$ $\log K_2$ at $\bar{n} = \dfrac{3}{2}$ and $\dfrac{1}{2} \log \beta$ at $\bar{n} = 1$ is obtained by extrapolation of formation curve. The value of $\log K_1$, $\log K_2$ and $\dfrac{1}{2} \log \beta$ are equal to corresponding p[A].

Observation and Calculation :

Room temperature: _______ °C.

Table 16.1

S. No.	Volume of 0.259 N NaOH added	pH of glycine hydrochloride mixture with sodium hydroxide	pH of glycine hydrochloride and copper complex mixture with sodium hydroxide
1.	0		
2.	1		
3.	2		
4.	3		
5.	4		
6.	5		
7.	6		
8.	7		
9.	8		

The value of ml of sodium hydroxide in X-axis to the corresponding value of pH in Y-axis can be extrapolated from the curve.

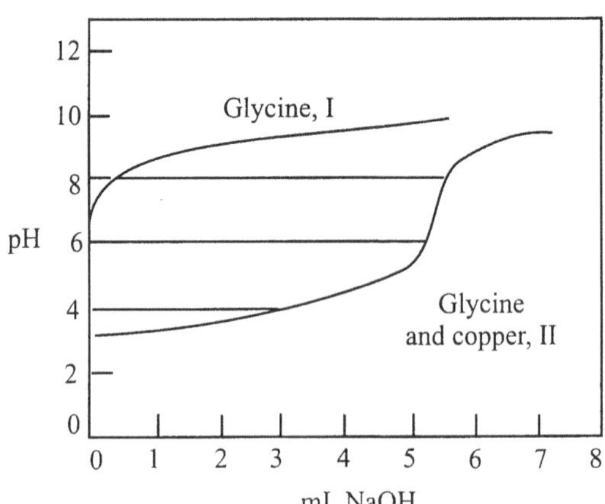

Table 16.2

pH	ml of NaOH solution per 75 ml sample	Total legand bound concentration	$\bar{n}$	p[A]
3.5				
4.0				
4.5				
5.0				
5.5				
6.0				
6.5				
7.0				
7.5				
8.0				

The volume of sodium hydroxide consumed per 75 ml sample can be converted to mole per litre unit.

[Let at pH 3.50 for 75 ml sample, 1.6 ml of sodium hydroxide is consumed. Then it (1.6ml) is in terms of mole/75 ml unit $= \dfrac{0.259\,M}{1000\,ml} \times 1.60\,ml$

$= 4.14 \times 10^{-4}$ mole, i.e., mole per 75 ml. Then, concentration in mole per litre

$= \dfrac{4.14 \times 10^{-4}\,mole}{75\,ml} \times 1000\,ml\ = 5.5 \times 10^{-3}$].

$$\bar{n} = \frac{5.5 \times 10^{-3}\,mole/litre}{9.45 \times 10^{-3}\,mole/litre} = 0.58$$

$$p[A] = pK_a - pH - \log\,([HA]_{in}\text{-}[Na\,OH]$$
$$= 9.69 - 3.5 - \log\,([3.34 \times 10^{-2}] - [5.5 \times 10^{-3}] = 7.6$$

From the formation curve at $\bar{n} = 1$, on extrapolation $p[A] = \dfrac{1}{2}\log \beta$ and β can be calculated.

Report : The stability constant of copper–glycine complex is ______ at ______ ^{o}C.

(**Note** : The log β value for this complex is around 15.3)

Questions and Answers

1. What are the importances of complexation?

   Ans :

   Metallic complex (chelation) :

   - Chelating agents and metal ion form water soluble compounds. EDTA, a chelating agent is used to remove metallic ions (calcium) from hard water.

   - *Drug Assay :* The assay of procainamide in injection is based on complex formation with cupric ion. The complex absorbs visible radiation. This is used as principle in spectrophotometry.

   Organic Complex :

   - Insoluble complex for masking taste – caffeine with gentisic acid.

   - Controlled dissolution: dissolution of caffeine in complex is slower than plain caffeine.

   - Effecting absorption and Bioavailability – Benzocaine and sodium salicylate complex: Benzocaine release is influenced. Release either increases or decreases depending upon ointment base.

   Polymer Complex :

   - Incompatibility of polyethylene glycols, polystyrene, carboxymethyl cellulose etc. – with certain drugs: physical, chemical and therapeutic incompatibility.

   - Polymer container and drug interaction: loss of active ingredients from liquid dosage forms.

   - Controlled release – prolonged action: useful in sustained release or controlled release delivery systems.

2. What is the unit of stability constant?

   Ans : It has no unit.

3. What are the other methods of determination of stability constant?

   Ans :

   - Method of continuous variations.
   - Solubility method.
   - Distribution method.
   - Spectroscopy etc.

17

Protein Binding

Many drugs are bound to plasma and tissue proteins. Though extent of protein binding is influenced by many factors, within certain dosage level it remains within a relatively small, more or less constant range. Chemical structure of the drug is the key parameter in protein binding.

Albumin is the main plasma protein involve in binding with drugs. Albumin concentration in plasma is about 4% w/v. Drug binding to plasma proteins occurs through ionic, Van der Waals, hydrogen, and/or hydrophobic bonds. The drug-protein binding is non-specific [many drugs bind to the same binding sites on the protein molecule. Being a reversible process, drug – protein binding can be expressed as

$$[D] + [P] \rightleftharpoons [D\text{-}P]$$

where D is drug and P is protein

Drug-protein binding influences:

- Distribution of the drug – bound drug (due to high mol weight of proteins) has restricted passage across capillaries and low lipid solubility prevents passage across cell membranes.

- Pharmacological actions (including side effects and toxicity) as the free (unbound) drug is only available for interacting with receptors, site of drug action.

The drug with higher affinity to binding proteins displaces a drug with lower affinity from its binding sites by competition. This increases the concentration of unbound drug of the latter (drug with less affinity). This has clinical significance only for highly protein bound drugs.

17.1 Determination of Extent of Protein Binding

Aim: To determine the extent of plasma protein binding of paracetamol at the end of 2 hours of incubation.

Principle: Drug and plasma protein (albumin) combine in a reversible way. The free (unbound) drug can only pass or cross a dialyzing membrane. The bound drug (drug-protein) complex can't cross the membrane.

When the drug and the protein are incubated at pH 7.4 biological buffer in a dialyzing membrane, the free drug can diffuse /pass through the membrane and diffusion continues both sides till equilibrium is reached. The measurement of concentration of the free drug at any point of time against a control provides the quantity of drug passed through the membrane.

The egg membrane can be used as dialyzing membrane.

Apparatus and materials required: Magnetic stirrer with thermostat, glass tubes (open at both ends), beakers, pipettes, egg membrane, egg albumin, paracetamol, phosphate buffer (pH7.4).

Process:

I. *Preparation of phosphate buffer of pH7.4:* 50ml of 0.2M potassium di-hydrogen phosphate (KH_2PO_4) and 39.1 ml of 0.2M sodium hydroxide (NaOH) are mixed and the volume is adjusted to 200 ml with distilled water.[Prepare 500ml buffer for this experiment].

II. *Separation of egg membrane:* A small perforation is made in the egg and the inner content is removed. Then the empty egg cell is placed in concentrated hydrochloric acid for about 3 minutes. With this hard cell gets dissolved and the egg membrane separates out. The membrane is washed thoroughly with distilled water to make it free from acid and finally equilibrated in buffer solution. The egg membrane is now ready for use.

III. *Apparatus setup:*

(i) The two glass tubes (open at both ends) specially made for this purpose are thoroughly cleaned.

(ii) One end of both the tubes is covered with egg membrane and tied.

(iii) The covered ends of both the tubes are dipped in phosphate buffer of pH 7.4 to maintain membrane activity. One tube is for test and the other tube is for control.

(iv) To Test tube: 1 ml of paracetamol (1%w/v) solution, 1 ml of phosphate buffer and 1 ml of egg albumin (10% w/v) aqueous solution are added.

Similarly to the control tube: 1 ml of paracetamol (1%w/v) solution, 1 ml of phosphate buffer and 1 ml of distilled water (solvent for egg albumin solution) are added.

(v) Both the tubes are immersed to the same extent as that of inside solution level, in two separate beakers containing 200 ml phosphate buffer. The contents of the beakers are kept stirred with the help of magnetic stirrer and the temperature is maintained at around 37°C.

(vi) At the end of 2 hours the concentrations of paracetamol in both the beakers are determined spectrophotometrically at 257 nm taking

$$A_{1cm}^{1\%} = 715 \text{ [for paracetamol]}.$$

The difference in the concentration between the test value and the control value can be used to calculate the extent of plasma protein binding at a given time.

Calculation:

From the absorbance reading, the concentration can be calculated using

$$A_{1cm}^{1\%} = 715$$

$$715 \text{ absorbance} = 1\%; \text{ x absorbance} = \left(\frac{1}{715} \times x\right)\%$$

As same amount of drug is kept in both tubes and dialyzed in same volume of liquid, the concentration ratio reflects the amount of substance ratio. Assuming equilibrium [the free drug concentration is same in inside and outside the dialyzing membrane],

$$\text{Percentage drug bound to protein} = \frac{C_c - C_t}{C_c} \times 100$$

Where C_c is free drug concentration in outside solution in control experiment and C_t is corresponding free drug concentration in test experiment.

Report: The extent of albumin (protein) binding of paracetamol at 2 hour is ————%.

Note: *The experiment should be continued till equilibrium is reached but it takes long time. The experiment is designed so that it can be conducted in regular practical class. However, it is suggested that to get the extent of protein binding, it is necessary to continue the experiment until equilibrium is reached.*

Questions and Answers

1. What are the other plasma proteins (other than albumin) responsible for protein binding of drugs?

   Ans : Though albumin is predominantly responsible for binding of drugs, α_1-acid glycoprotein (AAG) is also important in protein binding. Few common drugs which have significant binding to AAG are: Chlorpromazine, Diazepam, Haloperidol, and Quinidine.

2. What are the methods used for determining the extent of protein binding?

   Ans : Dialysis, Ultra Centrifugation, Ultra Filtration, Sephadexgel Filtration, Molecular Filtration, Electrophoresis, Agar Plate Method.

3. What are the clinical significances of extent of protein binding of drugs?

   Ans : When the degree of protein binding is high (more than 80%), the minor changes in the fraction of bound may produce relatively large changes in the proportion of unbound drug. When plasma albumin decreases (in case of malnutrition, liver diseases where synthesis is impaired or more albumin is lost), the fraction of bound drug is reduced. The fraction of free drug increased causing increased pharmacological action including toxicity. Reduction in AAG with pregnancy and with use of oral contraceptives may have similar situation. Excess pharmacological may arise from a reduction in the binding of some highly bound drugs like warfarin, phenytoin, valproate.

4. How is extent of protein binding expressed?

   Ans : It is expressed in terms of percent.

18

Rate Kinetics

18.1 Determination of Rate Constant

Aim : To determine the order and rate constant of reaction of acid catalysed hydrolysis of methyl acetate.

Principle : The reaction of acid catalysed hydrolysis of methyl acetate is:

$$CH_3 COOCH_3 + H_2O \overset{H^+}{\Leftrightarrow} CH_3 COOH + CH_3 OH$$

The acid (hydrochloric acid) is not consumed in the reaction. Acetic acid is produced in the reaction. The kinetics of the hydrolytic reaction can be followed by measuring the formation of acetic acid in the mixture, which can in turn be determined by withdrawing measured samples and titrating with standard alkali at time intervals and at the end of reaction.

The titre value is equivalent to the sum of the acid used as catalyst and acetic acid produced in the reaction. The difference of titre value at any time after the commencement of reaction and that at the commencement give the quantity of acetic acid formed, and the amount of methyl acetate hydrolyzed at that instant.

Apparatus and materials required : Thermostat, methyl acetate, conical flasks, pipettes, stop watch, standard M/2 hydrochloric acid, standard M/10 sodium hydroxide and phenolphthalein.

Process :

   (i)   A 250 ml dry conical flask containing 100 ml M/2 hydrochloric acid is clamped or placed in a thermostat maintained at 35°C.

   (ii) Around 15 ml methyl acetate taken in a clean and stoppered test tube is suspended in the same thermostat to attain thermostat temperature.

(iii) Five 250 ml conical flasks are filled each with 25 ml of water and some pieces of ice.

(iv) 5 ml of the ester is pipetted out into the conical flask containing acid and is mixed by shaking. Immediately (at zero time), 5 ml of the reaction mixture is pipetted out into the conical flask containing ice-cold water and titrated the mixture immediately with M/10 sodium hydroxide using phenolphthalein as indicator.

(v) Similar titrations are carried out by taking 5 ml samples at successive intervals of 5, 10, 30, 40 and 60 minutes. (Titre value gives the indication of amount of hydrochloric acid and formed acetic acid in the sample).

(vi) The remaining reaction mixture, with cork loosely fit, is placed on a water bath at around 50°C for at least one hour to complete the reaction. After cooling the mixture, 5 ml sample is withdrawn and titrated with M/10 sodium hydroxide as before.

Observation and Calculation :

Temperature of experiment : _______ °C.

Time in minutes	Titre reading in ml Volume of M/10 sodium hydroxide required to neutralize 5 ml reaction mixture	Acetate rémaining in the reaction mixture (volume of M/10 sodium hydroxide equivalent to amount of acetic acid formed) $(y_\infty - y_t)$	Concentration of acetic acid in the mixture = concentration of methyl acetate undergone hydrolysis (y_t)
0	x_0		
5			
10			
30			
40			
60			
t∞ (2 hr)	x_∞		

The initial concentration of methyl acetate can be calculated from the final titre value where methyl acetate is completely hydrolyzed.

Titre value at any point is the sum equivalent of hydrochloric acid and hydrolyzed acetic acid. Titre value at any point – (titre value at 0 time) is equivalent to amount of acetic acid.

Concentration of hydrolyzed acetic acid in the mixture is the indication of concentration of methyl acetate in the mixture.

1000 ml M sodium hydroxide 1000 ml M acetic acid = 1 M acetic acid

1 ml of used sodium hydroxide = $(1/1000 \times$ Strength of sodium hydroxide) M acetic acid

Let the titre value at time 0 (zero) = x_0

Titre value at any time t = x_t

Then, volume of sodium hydroxide required to neutralize the acetic acid formed at any time = $x_t - x_0$

At any time t, the concentration of acetic acid in the reaction mixture

$= \dfrac{x_t - x_0}{1000} \times$ Strength of sodium hydroxide = Lets say y_t M acetic acid.

The increase in acid concentration is a direct measure of amount of ester hydrolysed. At any time t, y_t mole of methyl acetate is hydrolysed.

1 mole of methyl acetate produces 1 mole of acetic acid.

[The initial concentration of methyl acetate – final concentration of acetic acid (where methyl acetate completely hydrolysed)]

$= \dfrac{x_\infty - x_0}{1000} \times$ Strength of sodium hydroxide $= y_\infty$ M acetic acid.

At any point of time t, amount of methyl acetate remained unhydrolysed $= y_\infty - y_t$

The plot of methyl acetate remaining Vs Time will confirm the order of reaction.

The reaction constant can be calculated from the slope of the curve (Log concentration remaining Vs Time, $-k/2.303$) or from the first order reaction equation:

$$k = \frac{2.303}{t} \log \frac{\text{Initial Concentration}\,(y_\infty)}{\text{Concentration at } t\,(y_\infty - y_t)}$$

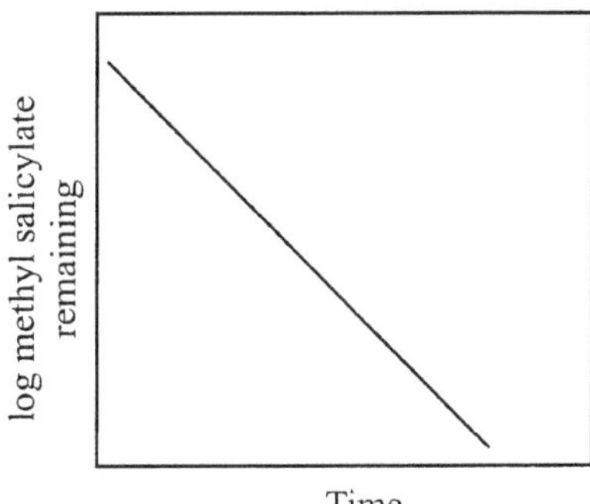

Report : The acid catalysed methyl acetate hydrolysis follows _______ order kinetics. The hydrolytic rate constant is found to be _______ /min.

(This reaction is actually pseudo first order as hydrochloric acid & water are in great excess).

Questions and Answers

1. What are the other methods of determinations of order of reaction?

   Ans : Substitution method is an alternative to graphical method (used in this experiment) to determine the order of reaction. The data obtained can be put into the rate equation and rate constant is calculated. When the rate constant value calculated k value remains constant within the limits of experimental variation, the reaction would be of that order.

   Zero order reaction: $k_0 = \dfrac{C_0 - C_t}{t}$

   First order reaction:

   $k = \dfrac{2.303}{t} \log \dfrac{C_0}{C_t}$

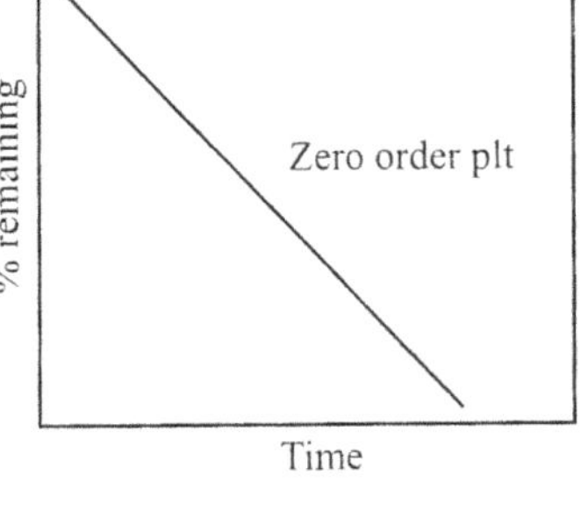

   Half life method can also be used.

2. What is the reason of adding reaction mixture to ice cold water?

   Ans : The reaction is stopped by bringing down the temperature using ice-cold water before analyzing the extent of reaction. The analysis should be carried out as soon as possible.

3. What are the importances of order of reaction or reaction kinetics?

   Ans : Order of reaction or reaction kinetics helps in determining the shelf life of products thus fixing the expiry date.

4. What is the unit of rate constant?

   Ans : The most of the pharmaceuticals under go degradation follow either zero order or first order reaction kinetics.

   The unit of k_0 (zero order constant) = moles/liter. second

   The unit of k (first order constant) = second^{-1}.

19

Stability Testing

A pharmaceutical product needs to be physically, chemically, therapeutically, toxicologically and microbiologically stable throughout its shelf life. The pharmaceutical companies do stability testing for estimating the shelf life and based on this the expiry date is given for the product.

The real time studies (long term testing) at recommended storage condition are ideal method for predicting shelf life. Often the studies are designed to increase the rate of chemical degradation or physical change of pharmaceutical products by using exaggerated storage conditions. This is known as accelerated stability testing. The pharmaceutical products are subjected to higher temperature and humidity conditions for accelerating the degradation. However, the results of accelerated testing are not always predictive of physical changes and potency.

The Pharmacopoeia specifies certain storage conditions. The Indian Pharmacopoeia (2010) defines the storage conditions by the following terms (replacing the earlier terminology like cold, cool, warm and excessive heat):

- Store in a dry, well ventilated place at a temperature not exceeding 30°C.
- Store in a refrigerator (2°C to 8°C). Do not freeze.
- Store in a freezer (–2°C to –18°C)
- Store in a deep freezer (below –18°C)

19.1 Accelerated Stability Testing based on Arrhenius Principle

Aim : To determine the shelf life of the product if stored at 25°C from the given data.

Principle : Though the medicinal products need to be physically, chemically, therapeutically, microbiologically and toxicologically stable, the chemical instability is most often the main consideration for determining the shelf life or expiry date. The medicinal products are stored at higher temperature condition to accelerate the degradation rate. This is known as accelerated stability testing. The rate of chemical reaction increases by 2 to 3 folds for every 10 °C rise in temperature in the region of room temperature.

The Arrhenius plot (log k Vs 1/T) from the equation: log k = log A – E/2.303 RT; (where k = reaction rate constant, R is the gas constant, T is absolute temperature and E is energy of activation) is used to find out the reaction rate constant at 25°C (desired storage condition).

The value of k is then placed in reaction equation to calculate $t_{90\%}$ (shelf life).

Following data are obtained from a study: drug products were kept at 55°C, 45°C and 37°C and drug content was analysed at different intervals.

Storage period month(s)	Potency retained at 55°C (mg)	Potency retained at in 45°C (mg)	Potency retained at 37°C (mg)
0	100	100	100
2	65	90	96
3	50	82	93
4	40	78	90
6	25	68	88

Materials required : Graph paper and calculator.

Procedure :

(i)   The order of drug decomposition reaction is determined first by plotting curve: Percent potency retained Vs time. (First order if straight line in semi log plot and zero order if straight line in Cartesian graph). Here it is first order.

(ii) The k value (rate constant) is determined for each temperature curve.

(iii) The Arrhenius plot is drawn: log k Vs 1/T.

(iv) The k value at desired temperature (25°C) is determined by extrapolating Arrhenius plot.

(v)   The value of k is placed in the first order rate equation and $t_{90\%}$ is calculated.

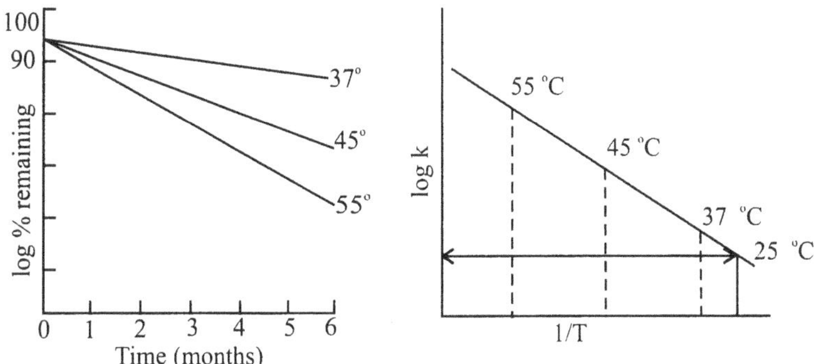

Calculation : The k value for 55 °C curve is:

$$\text{Slope} = -k/2.303 = \frac{\log 40 - \log 25}{4 - 6} = \frac{0.204}{-2} = -0.10$$

$$k = 0.235/\text{month}$$

Similarly the value of k for 45 °C curve is 0.068/month and the value of k for 37 °C is 0.011/month.

1/T value for 55 °C = 1/(55 + 273) = 3.048×10^{-3},

1/T value for 45 °C = 1/(45 + 273) = 3.144×10^{-3},

1/T value for 37 °C = 1/(37 + 273) = 3.225×10^{-3}, and

1/T value for 25 °C = 1/(25 + 273) = 3.355×10^{-3},

1/T factor is multiplied by 10^6 to get whole number (rather than fraction) for easy plotting.

The k value obtained by extrapolation of log k Vs 1/T curve at 25 °C is 0.003/month.

First order reaction equation : $\log C = \log C_0 - \dfrac{k\,t}{2.303}$

where C = potency at time t and C_0 is the potency at time zero.

$$t_{90\%} = \frac{\log 100 - \log 90}{0.003/\text{month}} \times 2.303 = 35.12 \text{ months.}$$

Report : The shelf life of the medicinal product is 35.12 months if stored at 25 °C.

Questions and Answers

1. Define the terms: Shelf life, Expiry date and Accelerated stability test.

   Ans :

   Shelf life : The period of time during which a medicinal product, if stored correctly, is expected to comply with product standard. It is used to establish the expiry date.

   Expiry date : The date mentioned usually on the label of the product up to and including which the product is expected to remain within product's standard (specification), if stored correctly.

   Accelerated stability tests : Studies designed to increase the rate of chemical degradation or physical change of a drug by using exaggerated storage condition. The obtained data together with real time stability data helps in assessing the stability of products and calculating the shelf life. They are not substitute of real time testing.

2. What are the other methods of predicting shelf life?

   Ans :

   (i) *Drawing of a plot :* Percent potency remaining Vs time for different temperature condition.

   (ii) Calculating $t_{90\%}$ for each temperature curve.

   (iii) Drawing $t_{90\%}$ Vs 1/T curve.

   (iv) Extrapolating the curve to 1/T corresponding to 25°C to get $t_{90\%}$.

3. How can the shelf life be determined from real time data?

   Ans :

   (i) Determining the order of decomposition. Zero order / first order (as most of pharmaceuticals degrade either by zero or first order)

   (ii) Calculating the degradation rate constant from the equation.

   (iii) Substituting the rate constant value in equation:

   (a) $$t_{90\%} = \frac{\log 100 - \log 90}{\text{degradation rate constant}} \times 2.303$$

   (first order process);

   (b) $$t_{90\%} = \frac{100 - 90}{\text{Degradation rate constant}} \text{ (zero order process)}$$

4. What should be the overage needed (in the above data) to get at least 5 years shelf life?

    Ans : In this case t = 60 months, the value of C = 90, k = 0.003/ month and the value of C_0 needs to be determined.

    $$\log C_0 = \log C + \frac{k\,t}{2.303} = 1.95 + 0.078 = 2.028,$$

    C_0 = anti log of 2.028 = 106.7 mg.

    The overage required is 6.7 mg.

5. Is $t_{90\%}$ always acceptable as shelf life?

    Ans : No. It depends on standard required for individual product (lower limit of acceptability).

19.2   Accelerated Stability Testing based on ICH Guidelines

Aim : To select the best formulation among the three products developed based on given stability study data.

Principle : ICH (International Conference on Harmonization for Technical Requirements for Registration of Pharmaceuticals for Human Use) guidelines recommend that the pharmaceutical products(drug products) should be subjected to 40 ± 2°C/ 75%RH ± 5% RH for 6 months for assessing the stability as a part of accelerated stability testing. In a six months study, a minimum testing frequency of 3 times: 0, 3 and 6 months is recommended. Accelerated stability testing aims at selecting the best formulation and container – closure system during development stage.

Following data are obtained from a study :

Three drug products were kept at 40 ± 2°C / 75% RH ± 5% RH and drug content was analyzed at different intervals.

Storage period in month(s)	Potency retained Product I	Potency retained Product II	Potency retained Product III
0	100	100	100
3	94.0	99.0	96.0
6	87.5	98.0	92.5

Materials required : Graph paper and calculator.

Procedure :

(i) The order of drug decomposition reaction is determined first by plotting curve: Percent   potency retained Vs time. (First order if straight line in semi log plot and zero order if straight line in Cartesian graph). Here it is zero order.

(ii) The k value (rate constant) is determined for all three products.

(iii) The product with the least k value is the best product.

Calculation :

The k value for product I :

$$\text{Slope} = -k = \frac{100 - 94}{0 - 3} = \frac{6}{-3} = -2$$

$$k = 2\%/\text{month}$$

Report : The best product is product _______.

Questions and Answers

1. What are ICH guidelines?

    Ans : ICH (International Conference on Harmonization for Technical Requirements for Registration of Pharmaceuticals for Human Use), a global agency, developed a series of guidelines on drug safety, efficacy, and quality that are acceptable in EU, Japan and USA. Stability testing guidelines are part of quality topics.

2. When ICH belongs to EU, Japan and USA, why are we interested on ICH guidelines?

    Ans : In world's pharmaceutical market, 75% of consumption (in terms of monetary value) is in these areas. Hence the pharmaceutical companies are interested to market their products in ICH countries. That is why we are interested on ICH guidelines as the data pertaining to safety, efficacy and quality are to be submitted based on ICH guidelines for obtaining marketing authorization.

3. When overages are permitted and when not permitted?
    Ans: In general, the overages are discouraged or not permitted in pharmaceutical products. They are not acceptable in case of potential hazards from over dose of newly made product or a toxic hazard from the degraded product at the end of the shelf life. Overages usually vary between 5 to 10%.
    As the little excess of vitamins do not have safety issues, the overages are usually permitted.

4. Is there any other method of calculating overage?
    Ans: From the plot of % potency retained Vs time, the $t_{90\%}$ is obtained. Then a line is drawn parallel to the line from the point of intersection of desired shelf life and corresponding % potency retained back to intersect the Y axis ['0' (zero) days]. The point at '0' time [Y intersect of the new line] should be the initial concentration required to get the desired shelf life. The difference between the extrapolated value at '0'time and the value at '0' of the original curve gives the % overage required.

20

Overages in Pharmaceutical Formulations

20.1 Determination of Overages in Pharmaceutical Formulations

Aim: To determine the overage required in the vitamin liquid formulation to get the shelf life of 1 year.

Principle: The overage is a fixed amount of drug added to a formulation in excess of label claim to compensate for degradation during the shelf life of the product. A minimum of shelf life period for medicinal product is necessary for viable marketing. In order to get this minimum shelf life, the overages are added to products like vitamin formulations.

The vitamins are very unstable substances and they degrade quickly. In order to have a product that would have the labeled potency at the end of shelf life, the addition of overages is necessary. The overage required can be calculated from the degradation rate equation. The equation for first order degradation:

$$\log C = \log C_0 - \frac{kt}{2.303}$$

where C = potency at time t,

C_0 = initial potency at time t = 0 (Label claim),

and k = degradation rate constant

The equation can be manipulated to get the desired initial potency, $^*C_0$, from the desired shelf life ($t_{90\%}$), C (at time t)). $t_{90\%}$ is usually accepted as shelf life.

The difference between calculated $^*C_0$ (desired initial potency) and C_0 (initial potency) is the overage required.

$$\text{Overage required} = {}^*C_0 - C_0$$

[Equation for zero order degradation: $C = C_0 - k_0 t$ Where C, C_0, and t stand for concentrations and time similar to first order equation; k_0 is zero order degradation rate constant.]

The following data are obtained from a real time stability data at 30°C:

Storage periods in months	Potency retained (%) /[This is also in mg][#]
0	100
3	94
6	90
12	78

Potency retained (%) and amount is same as the initial drug content is 100 mg.

Apparatus and materials required: Graph paper, scale, pencil, eraser and calculator

Procedure:

(i)   The order of drug degradation reaction is determined by plotting: % potency retained Vs time data in Cartesian as well as semi-log papers.

If the plot is linear in Cartesian paper the Order of the degradation Reaction is "Zero Order" and it is "First Order" if the plot is linear in Semi-Log paper.

[The data in the above table are of first order kinetics.]

(ii)   The k value is determined from the slope of semi-log plot.

(iii) The value of k is placed in the first order rate equation and $t_{90\%}$ is calculated.

(iv)   The $^*C_0$ for desired shelf life is calculated from the first order equation.

(v)   The difference between the calculated $^*C_0$ and the labeled potency gives the overage required.

Calculation: The k value for 30°C is

$$\text{Slope} = -\frac{k}{2.303} = \frac{\log 100 - \log 78}{0 - 12} = -0.01$$

Or, $k = 0.02$ /month

Now, it is necessary to calculate what should be the value of $^*C_0$ if it is desired to have the shelf life, $t_{90\%}$, for one year (or, 12 months).

$$\log {}^*C_0 = \log C + \frac{kt}{2.303} = \log 90 + \frac{0.02 \times 12}{2.303} = 1.95 + 0.10 = 2.05$$

$^*C_0$ = anti log of 2.05 = 112.20 [Equal to 112].

The drug content must be 112% of labeled potency when the product manufactured. In this case 112 mg of vitamin should be used in formula in place of 100 mg taking 12 mg as overage.

Report: The overage required for this liquid vitamin preparation is 12 mg [or, 12%].

Questions and Answers

1. What are the reasons for the addition of overages in pharmaceutical formulations?

   Ans: The overages are required to compensate foe degradation during manufacture or a product's shelf life, or to extend shelf life. There are two types of overages: Manufacturing overage and Stability overage. The manufacturing overage does not get reflected in the product label but recorded in manufacturing formula. The stability overage is justified based on drug degradation kinetics.

2. What are the issues for overages addition to the formula?

   Ans: The overage is not encouraged but is to be justified based on safety and efficacy of the product. The addition of overage may lead to super potency or toxicity and increased cost especially in expensive products.

3. When overages are permitted and when not permitted?

   Ans: In general, the overages are discouraged or not permitted in pharmaceutical products. They are not acceptable in case of potential hazards from over dose of newly made product or a toxic hazard from the degraded product at the end of the shelf life. Overages usually vary between 5 to 10%.

   As the little excess of vitamins do not have safety issues, the overages are usually permitted.

4. Is there any other method of calculating overage?

   Ans: From the plot of % potency retained Vs time, the $t_{90\%}$ is obtained. Then a line is drawn parallel to the line from the point of intersection of desired shelf life and corresponding % potency retained back to intersect the Y axis ['0' (zero) days]. The point at '0' time [Y intersect of the new line] should be the initial concentration required to get the desired shelf life. The difference between the extrapolated value at '0'time and the value at '0' of the original curve gives the % overage required.

Appendix

A.1   Best Fitting Straight Line

The use of straight line in defining the relationship of two variables: concentration Vs absorbance (in drug analysis), time Vs percent potency remaining (in kinetics of drug decomposition) and log k Vs 1/T (Arrhenius plot) is common in pharmaceutical science and practice. However, often we fail to get the straight line by joining all the points of an experimental observation. This could be due to poor experimental skill or incompetence or error in performing the experiments.

Examples of straight-line equations in pharmaceutical sciences :

$C = C_0 - k_0 t$ (straight-line equation of zero order process)

$$\log C = \log C_0 - \frac{kt}{2.303} \quad \text{(Straight-line equation of first order process)}$$

$$\log k = \log A - \frac{E}{2.303\,RT} \quad \text{(Arrhenius equation)}$$

The general equation of straight line is: $y = mx + c$

where y = dependent variable,

       x = independent variable,

       m = slope, and

       c = intercept in Y axis when $x = 0$.

When theoretically a linear relationship exists, but experimental observations do not fall on a straight line, it is important and desirable to draw a best fitting straight line. It is also known as trend line. As the best fitting line is based on least square method, the trend line is also called least square line.

If x_1, x_2, x_3 ——————, x_n and y_1, y_2, y_3 ——————, y_n are the data of an experimental observation; the slope $(m) = \dfrac{\sum (x - \bar{x})(y - \bar{y})}{\sum (x - \bar{x})^2}$

Intercept $(c) = \bar{y} - m\bar{x}$

To determine the value of slope (m) and intercept (c), the following calculations need to be done :

x	y	$(x - \bar{x})$	$(x - \bar{x})^2$	$(y - \bar{y})$	$(x - \bar{x})(y - \bar{y})$
x_1	y_1				
x_2	y_2				
x_n	y_n				
$\sum =$	$\sum =$	$\sum = 0$	$\sum =$	$\sum = 0$	$\sum =$
$\bar{x} =$	$\bar{y} =$				

Once the value of slope and intercept are determined, the corresponding value of y from respective value of x_1, x_2, x_3 ——————, x_n can be determined from the straight line equation. Then the straight line can be drawn using the new set of y values.

However, when it is necessary to have zero intercept like drawing the standard curve in drug concentration Vs absorbance relationship following Beer's law :

$$\text{Slope } (m) = \frac{\sum xy}{\sum x^2}$$

Note : However, it is always necessary first to determine whether or not the experimental data should fit into a straight line. In order to assess the same, it is required to calculate the correlation coefficient (r) from the given equation:

$$r = \frac{\sum(x - \bar{x})(y - \bar{y})}{\sqrt{\sum(x - \bar{x})^2 \cdot \sum(y - \bar{y})^2}}$$

when r = 1, there is perfect correlation exists and when r = 0, there is no correlation.

The value of r closer to 1, better acceptability of straight line.

A.2   Determination of Slope of a Straight Line

y = mx + c is the general equation of a straight line where m is the slope of the line and c is the intercept in y axis. The slope of a straight line is the ratio of change in y with corresponding change in x. i.e,

$$\text{Slope} = \frac{\text{change in y}}{\text{change in x}} = \frac{y_2 - y_1}{x_2 - x_1} = -k \text{ (rate constant in zero order)}$$

$$\text{Slope} = \frac{\log y_2 - \log y_1}{x_2 - x_1} = \frac{-k}{2.303} \text{ (rate constant in first order)}$$

A.3   Physical Constants of Water at different Temperature

Temperature (°C)	Density (kg/m³ × 10³)	Viscosity (mPa.s)	Surface Tension (N/m×10³)
20	0.998235	1.005	72.75
25	0.997073	0.8937	71.97
30	0.995674	0.8007	71.18
40	0.99224	0.6560	69.56
50	--------	0.5494	67.91

A.4   Sieve Number and Aperture Size

Sieve number	Sieve Size
5	4.00 mm
6	3.35 mm
7	2.80 mm
8	2.36 mm
10	2.00 mm
12	1.70 mm
14	1.40 mm
16	1.18 mm
18	1.00 mm
20	850 μm
25	710 μm
30	600 μm
35	500 μm
40	425 μm
45	355 μm
50	300 μm
60	250 μm
70	212 μm
80	180 μm
100	150 μm
120	125 μm
140	106 μm
170	90 μm
200	75 μm
230	63 μm
270	53 μm
325	45 μm

Bibliography

1. Patrick J. Sinko (2006), *Martin's Physical Pharmacy and Pharmaceutical Sciences*, B. I. Waverly Pvt. Ltd, New Delhi, Indian Reprint, 5ʰ edition.

2. R. Manavalan and C. Ramasamy (1995), *Physical Pharmaceutics*, Vignesh Publisher, Madras, 1st edition.

3. E.A. Rawlins (1975), *Bently's Text Book of Pharmaceutics*, ELBS and Churchill Livingstone.

4. M. E. Aulton (2002), *Pharmaceutics, The Science of Dosage Form Design*, Churchill Livingtone, 2nd edition.

5. S. J. Carter (1986), *Cooper and Gunn's Tutorial Pharmacy*, CBS Publishers and Distributors, New Delhi, 6th edition.